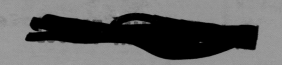

This Book Is In Memory Of

Carol
Tillotson Holmboe

(1941-1983)

Whose Special Expertise
Was Nurturing.

May It Help To Continue
Her Work Of
Caring and Sharing.

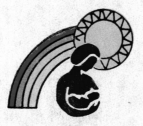

To my husband,
to my kids, to Val.
Thanks guys!
R.H.H.

To my parents.
M.E.

A NOTE TO THE READER
While writing and illustrating this book, we checked and rechecked the scientific information and the latest research. What we learned from scientists and health professionals is that knowledge about this subject is continually evolving and changing. While there is much agreement, there is also some disagreement, and some questions still remain. At this time, the information in this book is as up-to-date and as accurate as possible. If you have questions or need further information, you can check with your parents, doctor, nurse, health professional, teacher, or school counselor.

R.H.H. and M.E.
March 1994

LIBRARY OF CONGRESS CATALOGING-IN-PUBLICATION DATA
Harris, Robie H.
It's perfectly normal: Changing bodies, growing up sex, and sexual health / Robie H. Harris; illustrated by Michael Emberley.
Includes index.
ISBN 1-56402-199-8 (trade)—ISBN 1-56402-159-9 (pbk)
1. Sex instruction for children. 2. Sex instruction for teenagers. 3. Hygiene, Sexual—Juvenile literature. I. Emberley, Michael, ill. II. Title.
HQ53.H37 1994
613.9'07—dc20   93-48365

10 9 8 7 6 5 4 3 2 1

Printed in England

The pictures in this book were done in watercolor and pencil.
Book design by Lance Hidy

Candlewick Press
2067 Massachusetts Avenue
Cambridge, Massachusetts 02140

A Book
About
Changing
Bodies,
Growing Up,
Sex, and
Sexual
Health

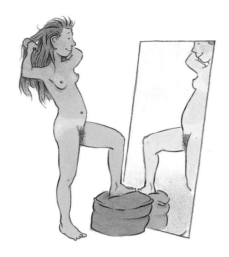

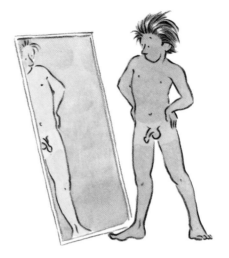

It's
Perfectly Normal

Robie H. Harris

illustrated by
Michael Emberley

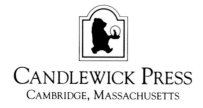

CANDLEWICK PRESS
CAMBRIDGE, MASSACHUSETTS

Contents

Part 4

Families and Babies

Part 5

Decisions

Part 6

Staying Healthy

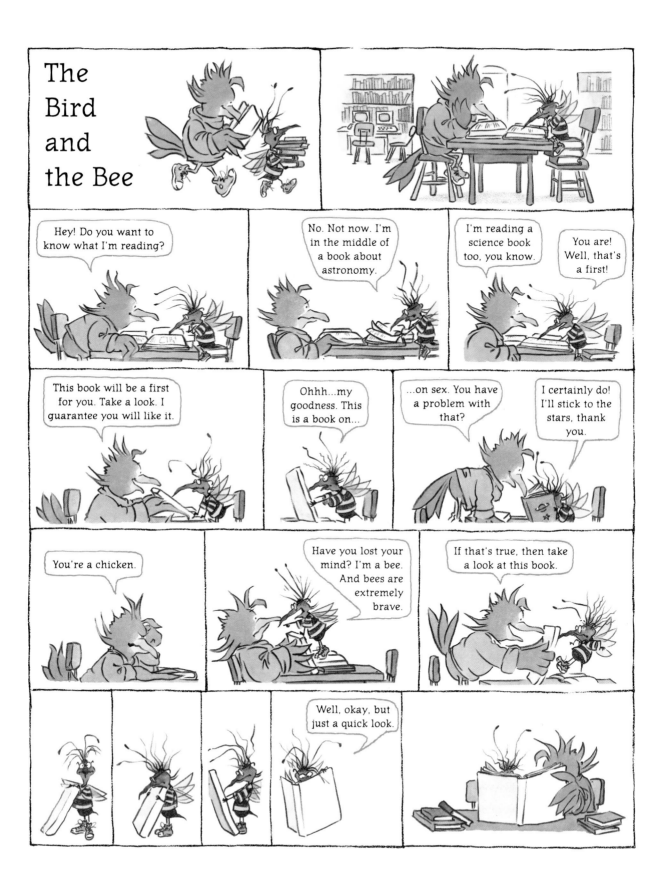

Introduction
Lots of Questions

Changing Bodies, Growing Up, Sex, and Sexual Health

Sometime between the ages of nine and fifteen, kids' bodies begin to change and grow into adult bodies.

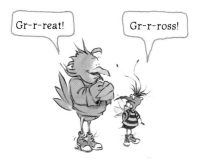

> Gr-r-reat!

> Gr-r-ross!

Most kids wonder about and have lots of questions about what will be happening to them as their bodies change and grow during this time.

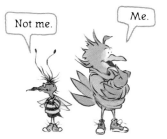

> Not me.

> Me.

It's perfectly normal for kids to be curious about and want to know about their changing and growing bodies. Most of the changes—but not all—that take place during this time make it possible for humans to make a baby and give birth to a baby. And making a baby has a lot to do with sex.

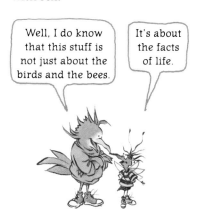

> Well, I do know that this stuff is not just about the birds and the bees.

> It's about the facts of life.

Sex is about a lot of things— bodies, growing up, families, babies, love, caring, curiosity, feelings, respect, responsibility, biology, and health. There are times when sickness and danger can be a part of sex, too.

Most kids wonder about and have lots of questions about sex. It's also perfectly normal to want to know about sex.

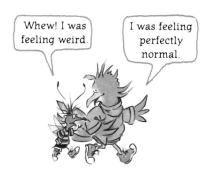

> Whew! I was feeling weird.

> I was feeling perfectly normal.

You may wonder why it's a good idea to learn some facts about bodies, about growing up, about sex, and about sexual health. It's important because these facts can help you stay healthy, take good care of yourself, and make good decisions about yourself as you are growing up and for the rest of your life.

Besides, learning about these things can be fascinating and fun.

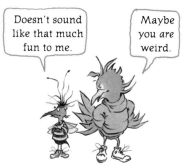

> Doesn't sound like that much fun to me.

> Maybe you *are* weird.

Part 1
What Is Sex?

1
Girl or Boy, Female or Male
Sex and Gender

What is sex? What is it... exactly? What is it all about?

These are questions lots of kids wonder about. You needn't feel embarrassed or stupid if you don't know the answers, because sex is not a simple matter.

Sex is many things, and people have many different feelings and opinions about it. That's why there is more than one answer to the question, what is sex?

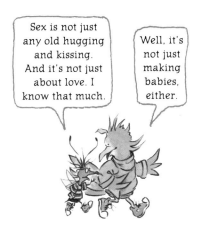

> Sex is not just any old hugging and kissing. And it's not just about love. I know that much.

> Well, it's not just making babies, either.

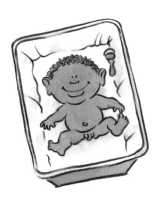

One way to find out about sex is to ask someone you know and trust. Remember, there are no stupid questions. Another way to find out about sex is to read about it. For example, you can look up the meaning of the word *sex* in the dictionary.

Here is what one dictionary says under the word *sex*:

1: *Either of the two main groups, female or male, into which living things are placed.*

People always want to know the sex of a new baby. So it's no

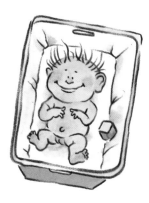

surprise that the moment a baby is born, someone always seems to shout out, "It's a GIRL!" or "It's a BOY!" And usually one of the first questions kids ask when they hear that a new kid is joining their class is, "Is it a girl or a boy?"

> Sex is in the dictionary!

> Think I'll head right over to the library.

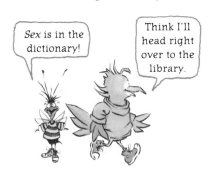

When people use the word *sex* in this way, they are usually talking about what gender someone is—whether a person is female or male, a girl or a boy, a woman or a man.

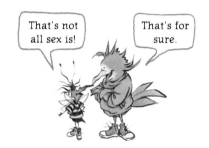

That's not all sex is!

That's for sure.

Gender is another word for whether a person is male or female. If a person is a boy or man, his gender is male. If a person is a girl or woman, her gender is female.

2
Making Babies
Sexual Reproduction

The dictionary tells us more about sex. It says,

2: *Sexual reproduction.*

Sex is also about reproduction—making babies. *To reproduce* means *to produce again,* or *make again.*

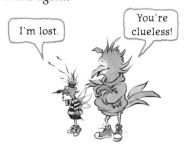

I'm lost.

You're clueless!

Certain parts of our bodies make it possible for a male and a female, when their bodies have grown up, to reproduce—to make babies. The parts of our bodies that make this possible are called the reproductive organs.

Our bodies' organs are the

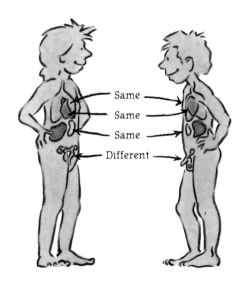

Same
Same
Same
Different

parts of our bodies that have special jobs to perform. For example, the heart is the organ whose special job is to pump blood. Scientists know that most organs inside our bodies, such as our heart, our lungs, and our stomachs, are the same whether we are male or female. One group of organs that is not the

same for a female and a male is the reproductive organs.

People also call the reproductive organs the sexual organs or the sex organs. The female and male sex organs are designed to work in an amazingly interesting way. They are different from each other because they have different jobs to do.

Both males and females have outer sex organs and inner sex organs. Some are located between our legs and are on the outside of our bodies. Some are tucked inside our bodies. The sex organs on the outside of a person's body are often called the genitals, and the sex organs on the inside of a person's body are called the reproductive organs.

If you are female, your vagina and ovaries are two of your sex organs. If you are male, your penis and testicles are two of your sex organs.

When the word *sex* is used in this way, people are usually talking about making a new human being—a baby.

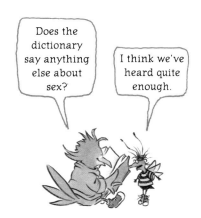

3
Strong Feelings
Sexual Desire

The dictionary tells us even more about sex. It says,
3: *Sexual desire.*

Sex is also about the desire to be physically close to someone, as close as you can be.

Do you ever really want or crave something? That's desire, like when you really want someone to be your best friend or when you really want chocolate ice cream.

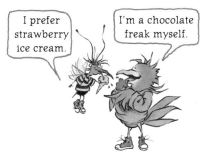

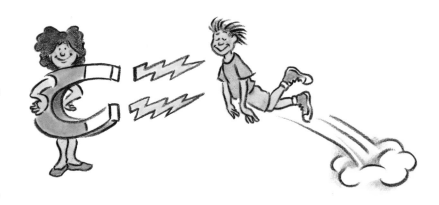

You don't know why you want these things. You don't even think about why you want them. You just want them. These are simply feelings of wanting—of desire.

Sexual desire is different from these desires—different from just wanting chocolate ice cream, or wanting someone to be your best friend, or even wanting to snuggle up to your mom or dad, a friend, a pet, or a stuffed animal.

Sexual desire means you feel attracted to someone in a very strong way...like being pulled by a magnet. You want to be as physically close to that person as you can be.

Even though you may think about that person a lot, sexual desire is mostly the way you feel in your body about that person. Your body may feel excited or warm or quivery or tingly. And sometimes these feelings can be very strong.

For lots of kids, part of sexual desire can be the fun of chasing and teasing or having a crush on someone. Often it's hard to stop thinking about that person, and you may even think you are in love with him or her. That's called "having a crush" on someone.

Both girls and boys have crushes. They have crushes on people they know, as well as on people they don't know—like TV stars, movie stars, rock stars, or sports stars.

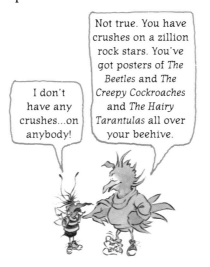

I don't have any crushes...on anybody!

Not true. You have crushes on a zillion rock stars. You've got posters of *The Beetles* and *The Creepy Cockroaches* and *The Hairy Tarantulas* all over your beehive.

They have crushes on people of the same sex, as well as on people of the opposite sex, on people who are the same age, older, or younger. Having a crush on someone is perfectly normal.

The feelings and thoughts you may have about other people and their bodies can make you feel very excited. Some people call this "feeling sexy."

Some of you are probably noticing the changes in your own bodies and the differences between your body and your friends' bodies. Sex can also be about the many new thoughts and feelings you may have about what's happening to you and your body as you are growing up.

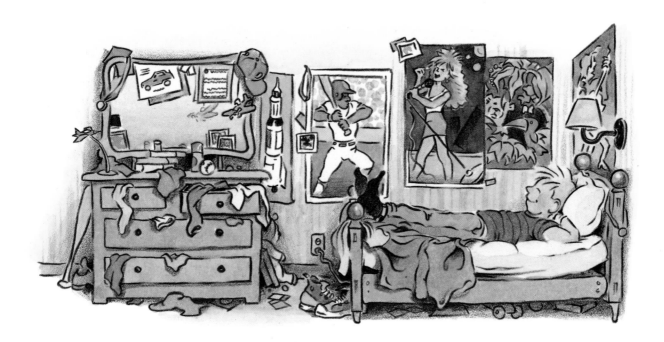

4
Making Love
Sexual Intercourse

The dictionary tells us one more thing about sex. It says, **4**: *Sexual intercourse.*

Sex also means sexual intercourse. Some people call sexual intercourse "having sex."

> Now we're getting to IT!
>
> Getting to WHAT?
>
> Oh, never mind. I wonder if you can find out even more about sex in the encyclopedia...

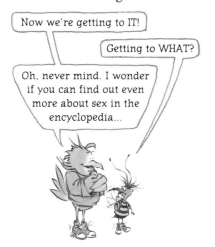

Sexual intercourse happens when a female and a male feel very sexy and very attracted to each other. They want to be very close to each other in a sexual way, so close that the male's penis goes inside the female's vagina. And the vagina stretches open in a way that fits around the penis.

When this happens, it is possible for a female and a male—

once their reproductive organs have grown up—to make a baby.

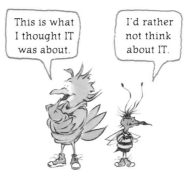

> This is what I thought IT was about.
>
> I'd rather not think about IT.

But most people don't have sexual intercourse only when they want to make a baby. Most often, they have sexual intercourse because it feels good. People

have sexual intercourse well into old age.

People also call sexual intercourse "making love" or "love-making" because it's a way of expressing love. But sexual intercourse is only one way of expressing love.

Hugging, cuddling, holding hands, kissing, and touching are other ways of expressing love. So is just being with someone you like a lot and telling that person, "I love you."

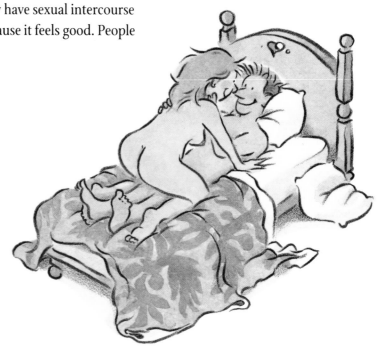

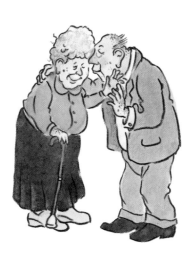

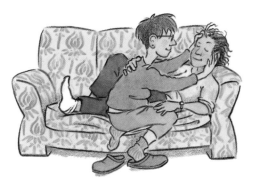

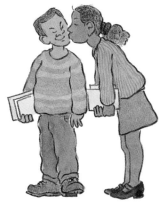

There are some things about sex and sexual intercourse that are important to know and remember:

- It makes good sense for a person to wait to have sexual intercourse until he or she is old enough and responsible enough.
- Every person always has the right to say no to any kind of sexual touching.
- A relationship that includes sexual contact often comes with complicated feelings.
- After sexual intercourse, the female can become pregnant. But there are ways that people can help protect themselves from having a baby.
- During sexual intercourse, serious infections—such as HIV, the virus that causes

AIDS—as well as other infections that are less serious can be passed from one person to the other. However, there are ways in which people can help protect themselves from getting or passing on these infections.

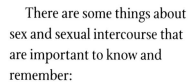

That's a lot to remember!

That's enough to remember.

So sex is a lot of things...even feelings...and thoughts.

Sex is the desire to be very close to someone.

Sex is intercourse.

Sex is making babies.

And sex is whether you are male or female.

Sometimes people use the word *sexuality* to talk about sex. When people use the word *sexuality*, they are usually talking about everything in our daily lives that makes us sexual human beings—our gender, our sexual feelings, thoughts, and desires, as well as any sexual contact, from sexual touching to sexual intercourse.

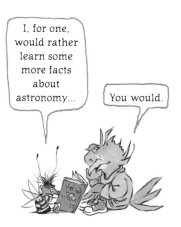

I, for one, would rather learn some more facts about astronomy...

You would.

5
Straight and Gay
Heterosexuality and Homosexuality

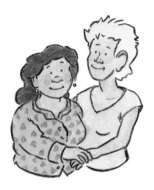 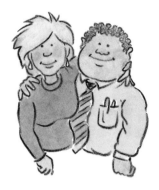 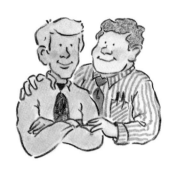

*S*traight and *gay* are two words that have to do with sexual desire and sex.

A straight or heterosexual person is someone who is sexually attracted to people of the other or opposite sex. *Heteros* is the ancient Greek word for *other.*

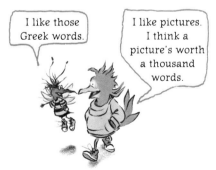

I like those Greek words.

I like pictures. I think a picture's worth a thousand words.

In a heterosexual relationship, two people of opposite sexes—a male and a female—may be attracted to, may fall in love with, or may have a sexual relationship with each other.

A gay or homosexual person is someone who is sexually attracted to people of the same sex. *Homos* is the ancient Greek word for *same.* In a homosexual relationship, two people of the same sex—a male and a male, or a female and a female—may be attracted to, may fall in love with, and may have a sexual relationship with each other.

A homosexual relationship between two females is also called a lesbian relationship. The word *lesbian* began to be used in the late nineteenth century. It refers to the time, about 600 B.C., when the great female poet Sappho lived on the Greek island of Lesbos. Sappho wrote about friendship and love between women.

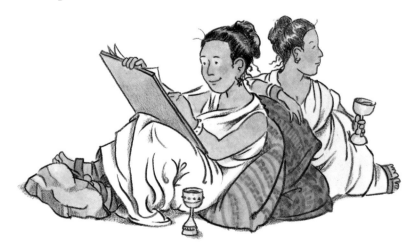

The ancient Greeks thought that love between two men was the highest form of love. In the ancient Greek city-state of Sparta, in about 1000 B.C., it was hoped that male lovers would be in the same army regiment. People thought that if a warrior was in the same regiment as his lover, he would fight harder in order to impress him. The Spartan army was one of the most powerful and feared armies in ancient Greece.

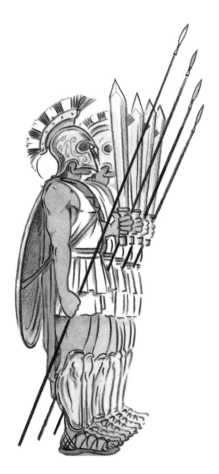

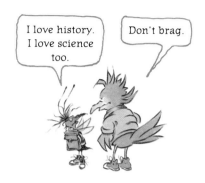

There have been gay relationships all through history, even before ancient Greece.

How people feel and think about homosexuality has a lot to do with the culture and the times in which they live.

Scientists do not completely understand or agree on why one person grows up to be homosexual and another person grows up to be heterosexual. In fact, there may be more than one reason.

Some scientists believe that being homosexual or heterosexual is not something you choose—just as you cannot choose what color skin you were born with or whether you were born male or female. They believe that a person is born with traits—with the biological makeup—that make him or her develop into a straight person or a gay person. Other scientists believe that events during a person's childhood help determine whether a person will grow up to be gay or straight.

Sometimes as kids are growing up, boys become curious about other boys and girls become curious about other girls. They may look at and even touch each other's bodies. This is a normal kind of exploring and does not have anything to do with whether a girl or a boy is or will be heterosexual or homosexual.

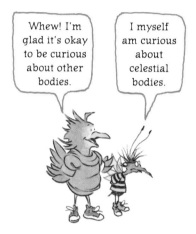

Dreaming about or having a crush on a person of the same sex also does not necessarily mean that a girl or a boy is or will be homosexual.

Some people disapprove of gay men and lesbian women. Some even hate homosexuals only because they are homosexual. People may feel this way toward homosexuals because they think homosexuals are different

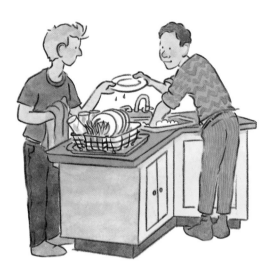

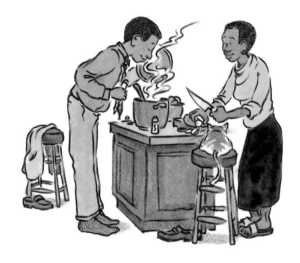

from them or that gay relationships are wrong. Usually these people know little or nothing about homosexuals, and their views are often based on fears or misinformation, not on facts. People are often afraid of things they know little or nothing about.

Some people are sexually attracted to people of the opposite sex and to people of the same sex. People who are attracted to, may fall in love with, and may have a sexual relationship with both males and females are called bisexual. *Bi* means *two*.

A person's daily life—making a home, having friends and fun, raising children, working, being in love—is, for the most part, the same whether he or she is heterosexual, homosexual, or bisexual.

If a person has any questions or thoughts about his or her sexual feelings, talking to someone he or she knows and trusts—a parent, a relative, a good friend, a teacher, a doctor, or a nurse—can be helpful.

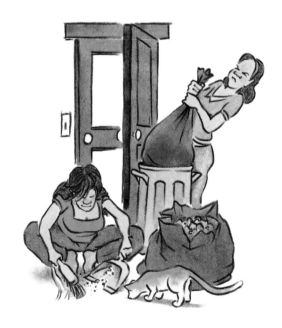

Part 2
Our Bodies

6
The Human Body
All Kinds of Bodies

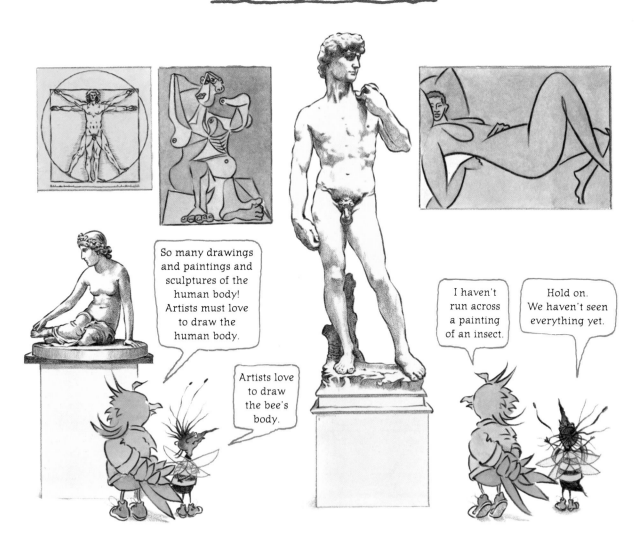

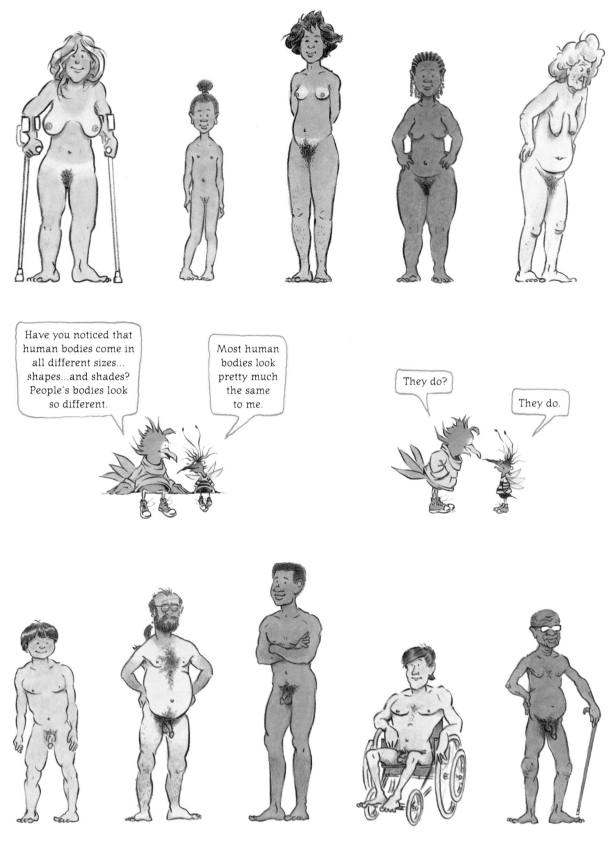

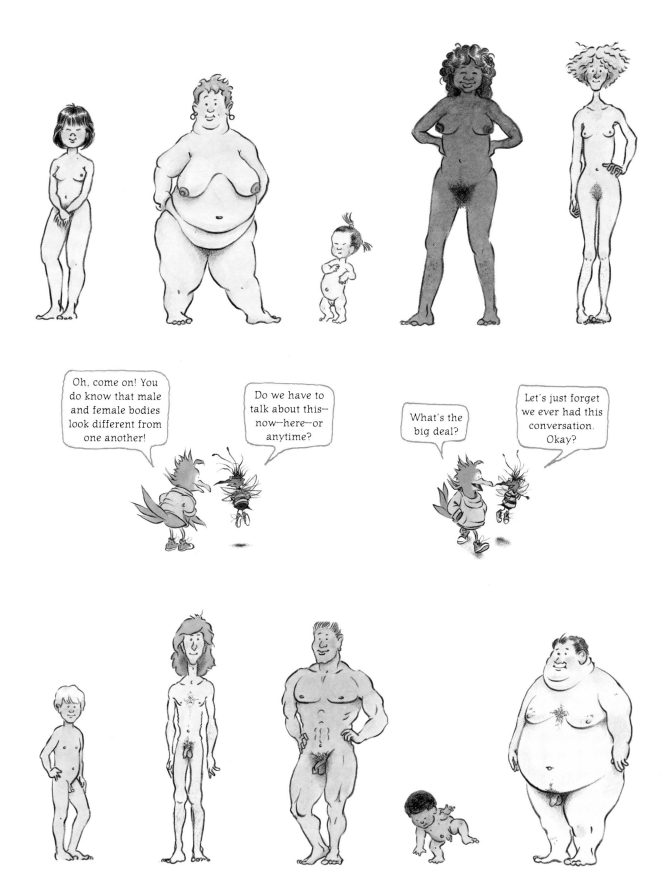

7
Outside and Inside
The Female Sex Organs

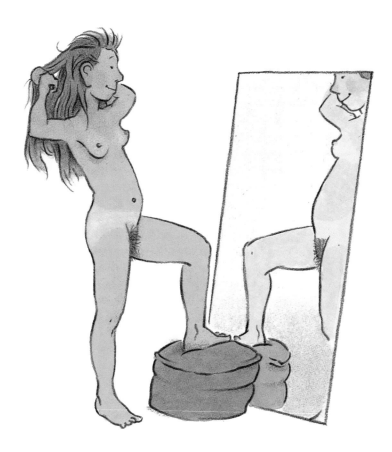

A female's outer sex organs, the clitoris and the opening to the vagina, are hard to see because they are located between her legs.

The Vulva
The whole area of soft skin between a female's legs is called the vulva. The word *vulva* comes from the Latin word *volva*, which means *covering*. The vulva covers the clitoris, the opening to the vagina, the opening to the urethra, and the labia.

The Labia
The labia are two sets of soft folds of skin inside the vulva. They cover the inner parts of the vulva—the clitoris, the opening to the urethra, and the opening to the vagina. *Labia* is the Latin word for *lips*.

The Clitoris
The clitoris is a small mound of skin about the size of a pea. When the clitoris is touched and rubbed, a female's body feels

good both outside and inside. It feels kind of tingly, kind of warm and nice. It feels sexy.

The Opening to the Urethra

The opening to the urethra is quite small. The urethra is not one of the female's sex organs. It is a tube through which urine—liquid waste—leaves the body.

BODY FACT: Urine is liquid waste from the body, liquid left over from food and drink that is not used by the body. Urine is the only fluid that travels through a female's urethra.

The Opening to the Vagina

The vagina is a passageway between the uterus—a sex organ inside the female body—and the outside of the female body. The opening to the vagina is bigger than the opening to the urethra.

BODY FACT: A thin piece of skin, called the hymen, covers part of the opening to the vagina. While a girl is growing—or when she is very active or during the first time she has sexual intercourse—the hymen stretches and may tear a bit, and the opening becomes somewhat larger.

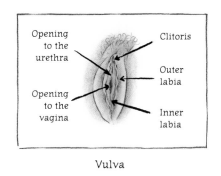

Vulva

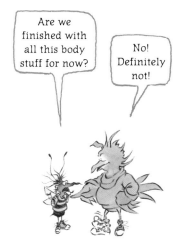

The Anus

The anus is a small opening through which feces—solid waste—leave a female's body.

BODY FACT: Solid waste is the solid material that is left over from food that is not used by the body. It leaves the female body in the same way that it leaves the male body. Solid waste is stored in the bowel before it leaves the body through the anus.

In all, from front to back, there are three openings between a female's legs: the opening to her urethra, the opening to her vagina, and her anus. If a girl or woman is curious about what these openings look like, she can hold a mirror between her legs and take a look.

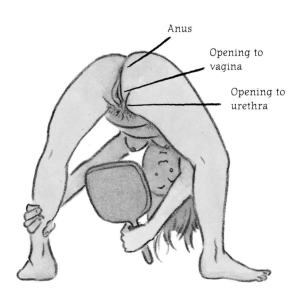

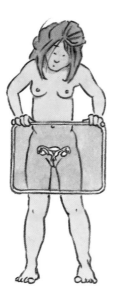

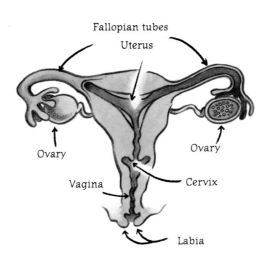

Fallopian tubes
Uterus
Ovary
Ovary
Vagina
Cervix
Labia

about the size and shape of a small upside-down pear and is connected to both Fallopian tubes and the inside end of the vagina.

Uterus

BODY FACT: The uterus is the place in which a developing baby, called a fetus, grows, is fed, and is protected. A fetus grows in the uterus, which stretches as the fetus grows bigger, for about nine months until it is ready to be born. The uterus is sometimes called the womb.

The Cervix

The cervix is a small opening located in the lower part of the uterus. It connects the uterus to the top of the vagina. This opening stretches wide when it's time for a baby to be born.

The Vagina

The vagina is the passageway from the uterus to the outside of the female body.

BODY FACT: A baby travels through the vagina when it is ready to be born. The vagina is also the passageway through which a small amount of blood, other fluids, and tissue leave the uterus, about once a month. This small amount of normal bleeding is called menstruation or "having a period" and begins when a girl has reached puberty. The vagina is also the place where the penis fits during sexual intercourse.

If you could actually look inside the female body and see the female's inner sex organs, you would see two ovaries, two Fallopian tubes, the uterus, and the vagina.

The Ovaries

The two ovaries—one on each side of the uterus—are about the size of large strawberries. The ovaries contain a female's sex cells—also called eggs or ova. A single egg is called an ovum.

Ovaries

BODY FACT: At birth, a baby girl's ovaries already contain an astonishing number of egg cells—about one to two million. But these egg cells are not grown up enough to produce babies until a girl begins to go through puberty. Puberty—the time when a girl's body starts to grow into a young woman's body—can begin anytime from about the age of nine until thirteen or fourteen. At puberty, a girl has about three hundred to four hundred thousand egg cells. A female's egg cells are no longer able to produce babies after the female is about fifty.

The Fallopian Tubes

The two Fallopian tubes are passageways through which an egg travels on its way to the uterus. One end of each tube almost touches an ovary. The other end of each tube is connected to the uterus. Each tube is about three inches long and the width of a soda straw.

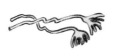

Fallopian tubes

The Uterus

The uterus is made of strong muscles and is hollow inside. It is

8
Outside and Inside
The Male Sex Organs

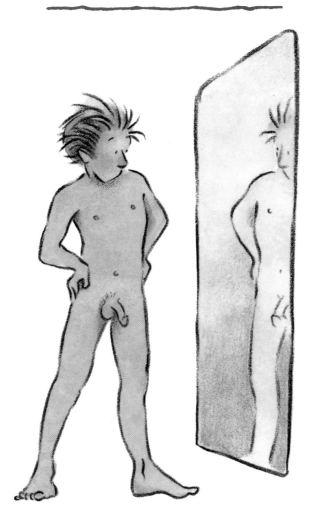

A male's outer sex organs, the penis and the scrotum—which contains the two testicles—are easy to see when a boy or man is naked because they hang between his legs.

The Scrotum

The scrotum is the soft sac of wrinkly skin that covers, holds, and protects the two plum-shaped testicles.

The Penis

The penis is made of soft, spongy tissue and blood vessels. Urine—liquid waste—leaves a male's body through a small opening at the tip of his penis.

The end of the penis is called the glans. When the penis is touched and rubbed, a male's body feels good both outside and inside—kind of tingly, kind of warm and nice. It feels sexy.

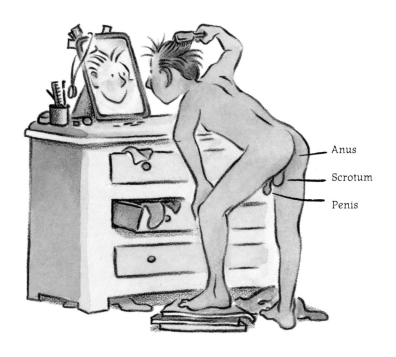

Anus

Scrotum

Penis

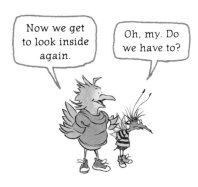

Now we get to look inside again.

Oh, my. Do we have to?

BODY FACT: Generally, the penis is soft and hangs down over the scrotum. Sometimes, it becomes stiff and hard, and larger and longer, and stands out from the body. This is called an erection.

BODY FACT: All males are born with some loose skin covering the end of the penis, called the foreskin. Some male babies have their foreskins removed a few days after they are born, by a doctor or a specially trained religious person. This is called circumcision. Although a circumcised penis looks different from an uncircumcised penis, both work in the same way and equally well.

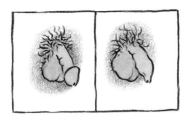

Circumcised penis   Uncircumcised penis

The Anus

The anus is a small opening through which feces—solid waste—leave a male's body.

BODY FACT: Solid waste is the solid material left over from food that is not used by the body. It leaves the male body in the same way that it leaves the female body—through the anus. Solid waste is stored in the bowel before it leaves the body through the anus.

In all, from front to back, there are two openings between a male's legs—the small opening at the tip of his penis and his anus.

If you could actually look inside the male body and see the male's inner sex organs, you would see two testicles and a series of tubes and glands that are connected to each other.

The Testicles

The two testicles are soft and squishy and are covered and protected by the scrotum. Usually one testicle hangs lower than the other. Before puberty each testicle is about the size of a marble. During puberty, each testicle grows to about the size of a walnut or a very small ball. That's why they are often called "nuts" or "balls."

Testicles

BODY FACT: A male's sex cells are produced in the testicles. Unlike female sex cells, which exist at birth, male sex cells are not made until a boy begins to go through puberty. Male puberty— the time when a boy's body starts to grow into a young man's body—can begin anytime from about the age of ten to about fifteen. At that time, a boy begins to produce sex cells. Male sex cells are called sperm, and males continue to make them into old age.

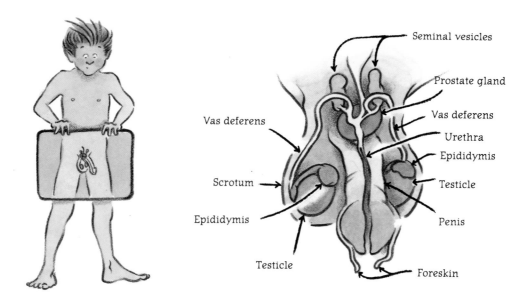

Seminal vesicles

Prostate gland

Vas deferens

Urethra

Epididymis

Vas deferens

Testicle

Scrotum

Penis

Epididymis

Testicle

Foreskin

The Epididymis

Each testicle is connected to its own small tubelike structure called the epididymis. Sperm travel through and "grow up" in the epididymis on their way to the vas deferens. Each epididymis is shaped like a telephone receiver but is much smaller.

Epididymis

BODY FACT: Each epididymis is a tightly coiled thin tube, which, if stretched out, would be about twenty feet long.

The Vas Deferens

The two vas deferens are each about a foot and a half long. Each of these long, narrow, flexible, and fairly straight tubes starts at the epididymis and winds all the way to the urethra. The two vas deferens are about as flexible as strands of cooked spaghetti.

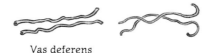

Vas deferens

BODY FACT: Sperm cells travel from each testicle through the epididymis and the vas deferens.

The Seminal Vesicles and the Prostate Gland

The two seminal vesicles and the prostate gland produce fluids that combine with the sperm to form a mixture called semen. *Semen* is the Latin word for *seed*. The sperm then travel along in the fluids to and through the urethra.

The Urethra

The urethra is a long, narrow tube that carries urine—liquid waste— from the bladder, where it is stored, to the penis and out through the opening at its tip. It is also the passageway through which semen leaves the male body.

BODY FACT: Urine is liquid waste from the body, liquid left over from the food and drink that is not used by the body.

BODY FACT: Semen, which carries a male's sperm, leaves a male's body in rapid spurts through the tip of his penis. This spurting is called ejaculation, and it occurs only after puberty has begun. Both semen and urine come out of the same opening at the tip of the penis. When a male ejaculates, muscles tighten and keep urine in his bladder so that urine does not leave the penis at the same time as semen.

9
Words
Talking about Bodies and Sex

Kids and grown-ups use all kinds of words for parts of the body and for sex. Some are scientific words. Some are unscientific—the common, everyday words that people use to talk about bodies and sex. Some of these words are nice, some are funny, and some are rude.

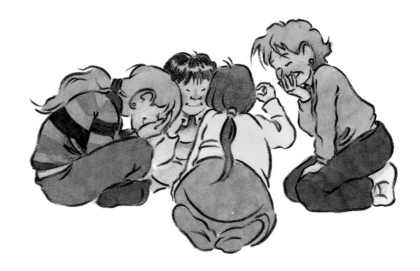

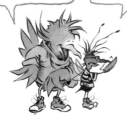

There are lots of silly-sounding words about sex and bodies—like "boobs" and "balls."

I much prefer the scientific words.

Everyday words are often called slang words. Rude and disrespectful words about sex and parts of the body are often called "dirty words." Jokes about bodies and sex are sometimes called "dirty jokes."

Some people think it's fun to use slang or dirty words and to joke about bodies and sex. Others feel embarrassed or uncomfortable when they hear these words. It's important to respect other people's feelings about slang and dirty words or dirty jokes, whatever those feelings may be.

Perhaps people feel uncomfortable talking about sex and bodies because we do not see our sexual body parts as much as we see our arms, legs, fingers, toes, ears, eyes, and noses. After all, our sexual body parts are usually covered by clothes.

Some people think it's wrong to think and talk or joke about bodies and sex. But many people think it can be comforting and helpful to talk about them with someone you know and trust like a friend, a parent, an older brother or sister, or a cousin.

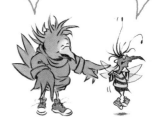

Did you ever notice that some grown-ups—not just kids—have a hard time talking about sex?

Yep! They twist around in their chairs and say "Well, uh..." about a hundred times or laugh nervously.

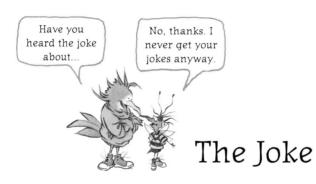

The Joke

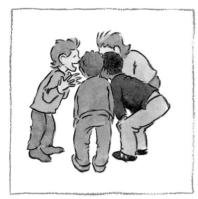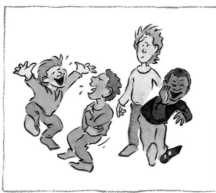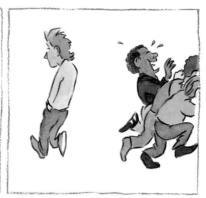

If you don't "get" the joke, you can always ask someone to explain it to you.

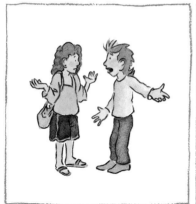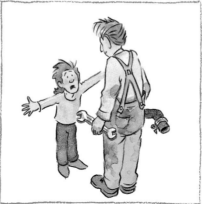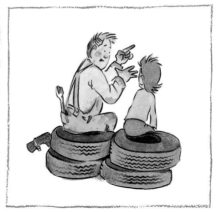

Part 3
Puberty

10
Changes and Messages
Puberty and Hormones

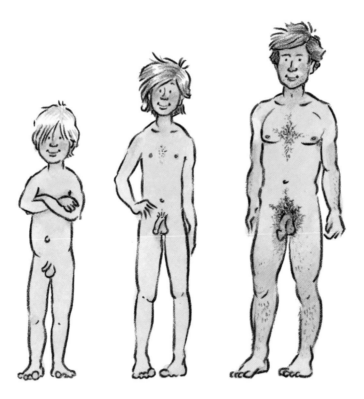

Our bodies change from the moment we are born and keep on changing all through our lives. They change because everything that's alive grows and changes.

But sometime between the ages of about nine and fifteen, girls and boys do more than just grow taller and bigger as they have done since birth. Girls start to grow into young women and

boys start to grow into young men.

Puberty is one of the names given to this span of time. The word *puberty* comes from the Latin word *pubertas,* which means *grown-up* or *adult*. When people use the word *puberty*, they are usually talking about all the physical changes that take place in kids' bodies during this time. Most of these changes make it physically possible for a female and a male to make a baby.

The other word that is used to describe the span of time between childhood and adulthood is *adolescence*. The word *adolescence* comes from the Latin word *adolescere*, which means *to grow up*. When people use the word *adolescence,* they are usually talking not only about the physical changes that take place during puberty, but also about all the new thoughts, feelings, relationships, and responsibilities kids have as they become young adults.

Even though the words *adolescence* and *puberty* have somewhat different meanings, people often use them interchangeably.

Puberty, or adolescence, is an in-between time—when a boy or girl is not a child anymore but is not yet an adult.

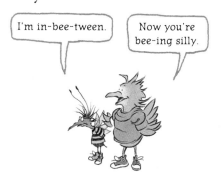

I'm in-bee-tween.

Now you're bee-ing silly.

Girls often start puberty when they are nine or ten or eleven years old. Boys often start puberty a year or so later—when they are ten or eleven or twelve. For most kids, puberty takes place over a stretch of time—over a few years. This usually gives kids time to get used to their adult bodies.

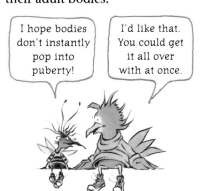

I hope bodies don't instantly pop into puberty!

I'd like that. You could get it all over with at once.

The many changes that take place in our bodies during puberty are caused by hormones. Hormones are chemicals that are produced in many different places in our bodies. Hormones travel through the body's bloodstream from the place where they are made to other places in the body where they do their work.

The word *hormone* comes from the Greek word *hormon,* meaning *to set in motion*—to start something working. There are many kinds of hormones in our bodies.

During puberty, the brain begins to manufacture special

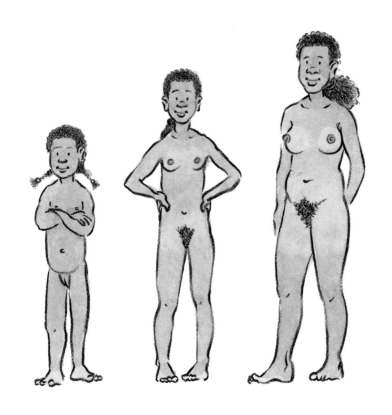

hormones. These hormones send a message to the sex organs—a boy's testicles or a girl's ovaries—that tells them to start working—to start producing sex hormones.

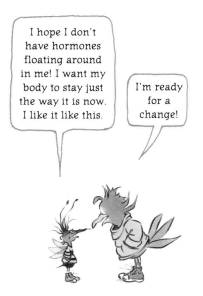

I hope I don't have hormones floating around in me! I want my body to stay just the way it is now. I like it like this.

I'm ready for a change!

The sex hormones in the male body then instruct the testicles to make sperm. The sex hormones in the female body then instruct the ovaries to send out an egg.

It is the sex hormones that cause the changes that make children's bodies grow into adult bodies. Only then is it possible for humans to have babies.

Once the sex hormones start working, puberty begins. Some sex hormones cause changes to take place in and around boys' and girls' sex organs. Others cause changes to take place throughout their bodies. Sex hormones can also affect girls' and boys' feelings and moods.

Many cultures, religions, com- munities, and families mark the beginning of puberty for a boy or girl with a celebration or ceremony. They view puberty as a special part of growing up. Others choose to let a boy or girl enter puberty without a celebration or ceremony. They view puberty simply as a regular and ordinary part of growing up.

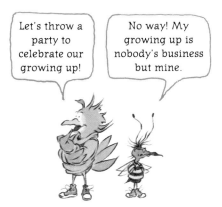

Let's throw a party to celebrate our growing up!

No way! My growing up is nobody's business but mine.

11
The Travels of the Egg
Female Puberty

"Start making female sex hormones!" is one of the messages the female's brain sends to her ovaries at puberty. And the ovaries do just that. They begin to produce the hormones estrogen and progesterone. Estrogen tells the eggs, which have been in a girl's ovaries since birth, to grow

up. Usually only one egg grows up at a time.

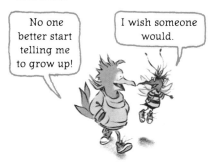

No one better start telling me to grow up!

I wish someone would.

When the eggs grow up, the ovaries do something they've never done before. About once a month, they begin to release a single grown-up egg. An egg is about the size of a grain of sand.

Eggs are female sex cells. A girl's ovaries usually begin releasing eggs during puberty. In her life, she will release about four hundred to five hundred eggs. The release of an egg is called ovulation. The word *ovulation* comes from the word *ovum*, meaning *egg*.

At about the same time every month, when an egg is released from one of the ovaries, it is swept by tiny fingerlike projections into one of the Fallopian tubes, where it begins its travels to the uterus.

The Fallopian tube is the place where an egg can meet and unite with a sperm. Once an egg has united with a sperm, they become the beginning cell of a baby. The uniting of an egg cell and a sperm cell is called conception or fertilization.

The fertilized egg continues to travel through the Fallopian tube and into the uterus, where the female sex hormone progesterone has helped to create a soft lining that is ready to receive it. The fertilized egg then plants itself in the lining of the uterus. This soft, thick, cozy lining is made of extra blood vessels, tissue, and other fluids and is created so that the fertilized egg will have a healthy place to grow.

If the egg has been fertilized, it will plant itself in the uterus and stay there—and grow into a baby. However, most of the time, the egg is not fertilized. If the egg

does not unite with a sperm within about twenty-four to thirty-six hours after leaving an ovary, it does not stay in the uterus and does not go on to develop into a baby.

Instead, the egg breaks down while it is in the uterus and mixes with some of the extra blood and fluid in the soft lining of the uterus. Since there is no fertilized egg starting to grow in the uterus, this soft lining is not needed and dissolves. It then passes out of the uterus, through the vagina, and out of the body in the form of a small amount of blood, other fluids, and tissue. The lining's monthly passing out of the uterus and the vagina is called menstruation. The word *menstruation* comes from the Latin word *mensis*, which means *month*.

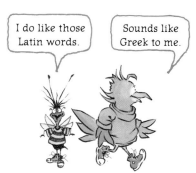

I do like those Latin words.

Sounds like Greek to me.

The period of time from the beginning of one menstruation to the next is about a month long and is called the menstrual cycle.

Girls usually start to menstruate after their ovaries have begun

to release eggs. As soon as a girl's ovaries have begun to release eggs, she can become pregnant if she has had sexual intercourse.

But some girls may begin to release eggs even before they start to menstruate. This means that it is possible, although quite rare, for a girl to become pregnant before she has started to menstruate. Girls usually start to menstruate at the age of eleven or twelve. But some start as early as age nine and others start as late as age fifteen, and that's perfectly normal.

The very first time a girl menstruates, she may worry that a large amount of blood will suddenly flow out. In fact, the blood usually comes out slowly. Only a few tablespoonfuls to about half a cup of blood and tissue dribble out during each menstruation. But the amount can be more or less, and that's also perfectly normal.

This dribbling continues over a period of a few days. That's why people call menstruation a menstrual period or "having your period." Other kids call menstruation "my friend," "that time of the month," or "the curse." No matter what people call it, menstruation is a healthy occurrence.

A period usually lasts about three to eight days. When a girl

THE TRAVELS OF THE EGG: *Menstruation*

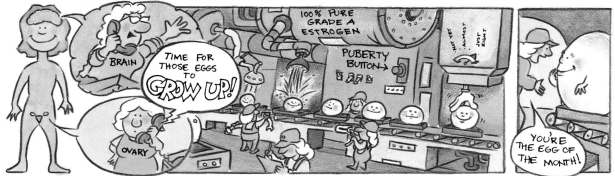

At puberty the brain tells the ovaries to produce estrogen, which tells the eggs to mature.

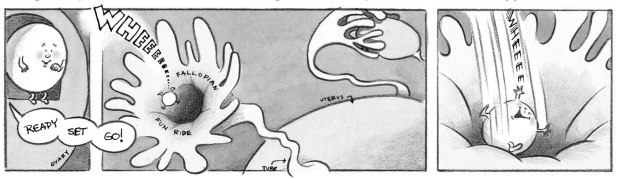

And then, about once a month, an egg leaves an ovary and pops into a Fallopian tube,

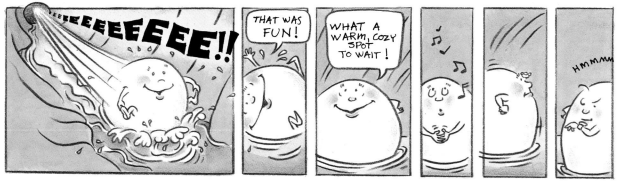

where it waits before traveling to the uterus.

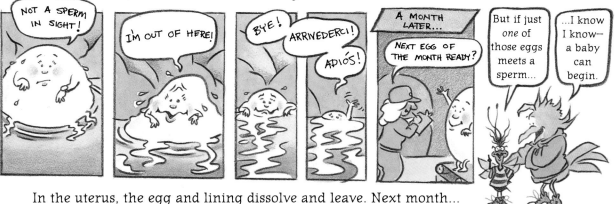

In the uterus, the egg and lining dissolve and leave. Next month...

first starts to menstruate, her periods often come irregularly—sometimes a few weeks apart, sometimes many weeks apart. It can often take up to one or two years for a girl's period to occur on a regular schedule—about once a month. Some women's and girls' periods never become regular, and that is perfectly normal too.

Most girls and women continue their regular activities during menstruation. For example, they bathe, shower, swim, play sports, dance, and do whatever they normally like to do. Some girls and women do get cramps—usually slight, tight pains around the area of the uterus—before and during their periods. Most cramps are normal.

When girls and women travel, play sports vigorously, lose or gain a lot of weight, or become upset or ill, their periods can become irregular for a while. And when a female becomes pregnant, her periods stop until after the baby is born.

When women are about fifty years old, their bodies start to make fewer sex hormones. As a result, their ovaries stop releasing eggs, and they stop menstruating. This period of time in a woman's life is called menopause—the pausing and stopping of menstruation. When a woman stops having menstrual periods, she is no longer able to become pregnant.

During a menstrual period, a girl or woman uses pads or tampons to absorb the menstrual

flow that passes out of her vagina so it will not leak on her underpants or other clothes. She can use whichever is more comfortable.

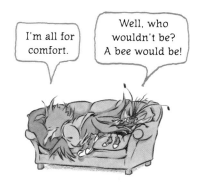

I'm all for comfort.

Well, who wouldn't be? A bee would be!

Pads are also called sanitary napkins. *Sanitary* means *clean.* Pads and tampons are made of a clean, soft, cottonlike material and absorb the menstrual flow. A pad fits on the inside of a girl or woman's underpants, just outside the opening to her vagina. Most

Where a Pad Fits

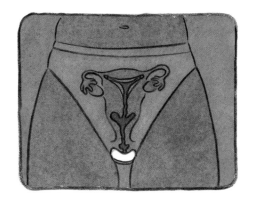

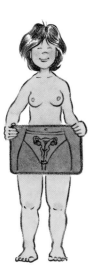

Pads

Where a Tampon Fits

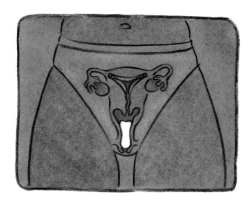

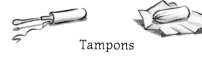

Tampons

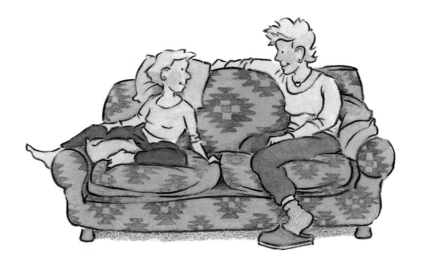

ready for her first period, where to get pads or tampons, and how to use them. This kind of information can help prepare a girl for her first period—whether it starts when she is at home or out with friends or in school. She may also want to carry a pad or tampon in her purse or knapsack in case she gets her first period when she is not at home.

No matter how well prepared she is, a girl's first period usually comes as somewhat of a surprise. For some girls, it may feel quite exciting; for others, a bit scary. But no matter how a girl feels, starting to menstruate is a perfectly normal and natural part of growing up. Most girls feel that starting to menstruate is one of the biggest changes of puberty.

pads come with a small piece of adhesive tape on one side that keeps the pad in place. Tampons fit inside the vagina. A tampon cannot move into the uterus because the cervix is too small an opening for a tampon to pass through.

One way a girl can find out when she might get her first period is to ask her mother. If her mother started menstruating early, there's a good chance she may start early too. If her mother started later, there's a good chance that she may start later.

Talking to someone about menstruation—one's mother or grandmother or aunt, or an older friend or cousin—can be helpful. A girl can find out many useful things from someone who is already menstruating, such as what it feels like to menstruate, what she will need to do to get

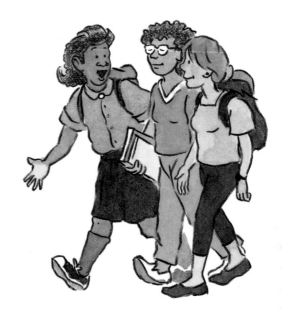

12
The Travels of the Sperm
Male Puberty

"Start making the male sex hormone testosterone!" is one of the messages a boy's brain sends out to his testicles during puberty. And the testicles do just that. They begin to produce testosterone, which causes the male body to grow and change in many new ways.

One of the most important things testosterone does is instruct the testicles to begin to make sperm—something the testicles have never done before.

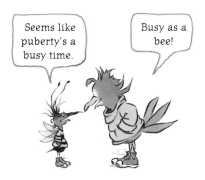

Seems like puberty's a busy time.

Busy as a bee!

Sperm are male sex cells. Unlike girls, boys do not start making sex cells until they reach puberty. Starting at puberty, however, the testicles make a phenomenal number of sperm—about one hundred million to three hundred million sperm per day. That's anywhere from about one thousand to three thousand sperm every second.

The scrotum protects the testicles by keeping them at the right temperature to make sperm, not too cold and not too hot, just a few degrees below the body's temperature. If it is too cold, the scrotum pulls up the testicles closer to the body to keep them warm enough to make sperm. When a man or boy is swimming in cold water, he can often feel his scrotum tighten as it pulls up his testicles. If it is too hot, the scrotum hangs down loosely, away from the body, again keeping the testicles at just the right temperature to make sperm.

After sperm are produced, the sperm from the right testicle travel through the right epididymis, and the sperm from the left testicle travel through the left epididymis. As they travel, the sperm grow up enough to be able to fertilize—to unite with—a female's egg.

Sperm travel through the vas deferens and pass by the seminal vesicles. As sperm pass by, they mix with fluid from the seminal vesicles and the prostate gland.

The mixture of sperm and fluid is now called semen. Semen is sticky, cloudy, and whitish. Chemicals in it keep the sperm healthy as they travel into the urethra, through it, and out the tip of the penis.

Sperm leave the male body when a male ejaculates semen. *To ejaculate* means *to suddenly release* or *to let go*. When a male ejaculates, his penis is usually erect.

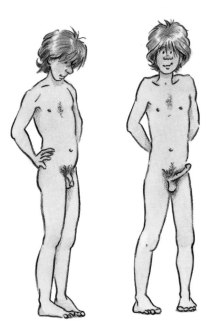

Here's what happens inside a male's body when he has an erec-

THE TRAVELS OF THE SPERM: *Ejaculation*

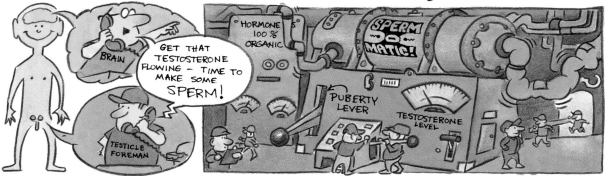

At puberty the brain tells the testicles to produce testosterone and sperm.

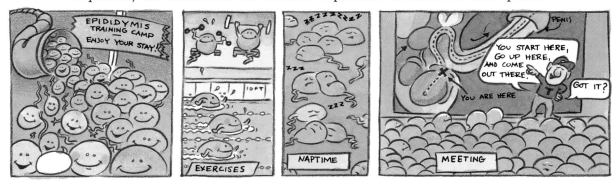

Sperm travel to the epididymis where they mature and travel

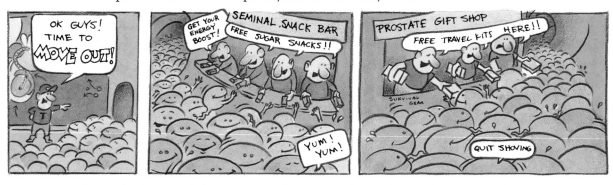

through the vas deferens, past the seminal vesicles and prostate gland,

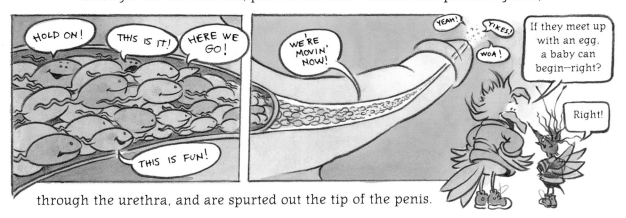

through the urethra, and are spurted out the tip of the penis.

tion: When his penis is not erect, blood trickles in and out of the penis continuously. But when he has an erection, the muscles that allow blood to flow in and out of his penis open wide and allow more blood to be pumped in, while other muscles tighten and keep the extra amount of blood from leaving the penis. This causes the spongy tissue inside the penis to fill up, which in turn makes the penis become stiff, erect, and stand out from the body. This filling up is called an erection.

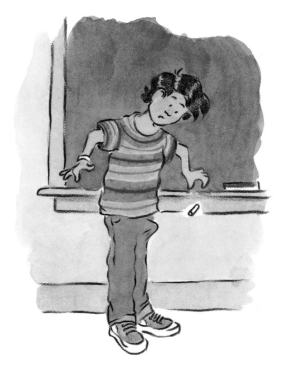

When the erection is over, the muscles relax and allow the blood to flow back out of the penis and into the body again. And the penis becomes soft again.

A male can have an erection when his penis is touched and rubbed; when he has pleasurable thoughts or sees someone who makes him feel happy, excited, sexy, or nervous; when he is watching a movie or TV show and something in the movie or on TV excites him; when someone attractive to him walks by; or when he is having a pleasurable dream.

Males often have erections when they wake up. If a male's bladder—the place where urine is stored in his body—is full, the full bladder excites some nerves at the base of his penis, which causes more blood to flow into the penis. This kind of erection has little to do with sexy thoughts and feelings.

Males usually have erections before and during sexual intercourse. An erection makes it possible for the penis to enter the vagina. Sometimes males have erections for no apparent reason, even when they don't want to have them.

Some people call an erection a "hard-on" or "boner" even though there are no bones in the penis. Erections usually last a few seconds, to a few minutes, to a half-hour, or more. Males can have erections from the time they are little babies until they are old men.

Here's what happens inside a male's body when he has an ejaculation: Muscles in each epididymis, in each vas deferens, and in the seminal vesicles, along with muscles around the prostate gland, tighten and push the semen into the urethra. The semen, which contains sperm, travels through the urethra and spurts out through the tip of the penis. This spurting out of semen—ejaculation—causes a feeling of excitement called an orgasm.

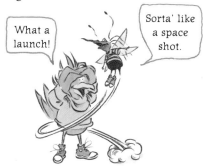

What a launch!

Sorta' like a space shot.

After ejaculation, the penis becomes soft again and is no longer erect.

There are usually about two to five hundred million sperm spurted out in a single ejaculation—about a teaspoonful of semen.

Males can and do have erections without ejaculating any semen. When this happens, the blood leaves the penis slowly and returns to the body's bloodstream, the erection slowly goes away, and the penis becomes soft again and hangs down as usual. It is also possible, although this does not happen very often, for a male to ejaculate without having an erection.

Boys start to be able to ejaculate during puberty and continue well into old age. Ejaculation usually occurs during sexual intercourse. It can also occur during other kinds of sexual touching and excitement and even during sleep.

Boys usually start having "wet dreams" at puberty. Wet dreams

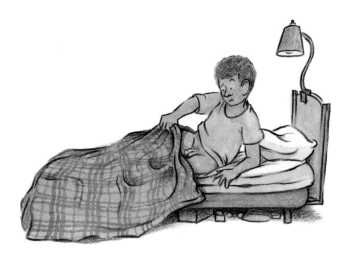

occur during sleep when a boy is having a pleasurable, exciting, or sexy dream and ejaculates some semen. When the boy wakes up, his pajamas or sheets may be wet and sticky from the ejaculated semen.

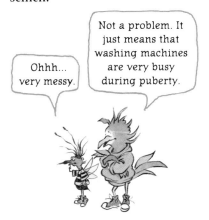

The scientific term for a wet dream is *nocturnal emission*. *Nocturnal* means *occuring at night*. *Emission* means *a release, a letting go*. Wet dreams are usual and normal events for boys. A boy's first ejaculation often happens during a dream.

Once a male has begun to produce sperm, if just one of his sperm unites with an egg during sexual intercourse, the female can become pregnant and the united cell can grow and develop into a baby.

Many boys feel that starting to ejaculate is one of the biggest changes of puberty.

13
Not All at Once!
Growing and Changing Bodies

During puberty, the sex hormones cause boys and girls to grow and change in even more ways.

All these changes do not take place at once. Most of them happen slowly over a few years' time; a few happen quickly. And they often, although not always, take place in a somewhat specific order.

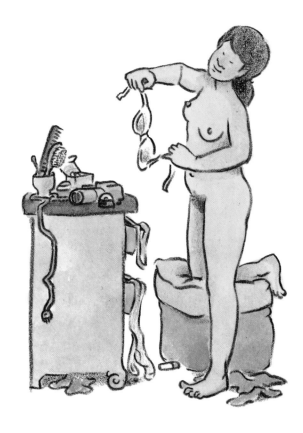

Girls: Puberty Changes

- Ovaries gradually grow larger.
- Body sweats more.
- Skin and hair become more oily.
- Body has a sudden growth spurt.
- Body gains some weight and grows taller.
- Arms and legs grow longer.
- Hands and feet grow bigger.
- Bones in the face grow larger and longer, and the face looks less childlike.
- Soft, darkish hair grows around the vulva and later becomes curly, thick, and coarse.
- A tiny bit of sticky whitish fluid may come out of the vagina.

PUBERTY FACT: The whitish fluid that may flow out of the vagina is normal and helps keep it clean and healthy.

- Hips grow wider. Body begins to look more curvy.

PUBERTY FACT: A girl's hips grow wider, so that if and when she decides to have a baby, her baby will have enough room to leave the uterus when it is ready to be born.

- Hair grows under the arms.
- Breasts and nipples gradually grow larger and fuller.

PUBERTY FACT: A girl's breasts grow larger and fuller to prepare her body to make milk to nurse her baby if and when she has one.

- Nipples may become a darker color.
- Menstruation can begin.

PUBERTY FACT: Once the ovaries have grown larger, they start to release grown-up eggs, and menstruation begins. Once menstruation starts, a girl can become pregnant.

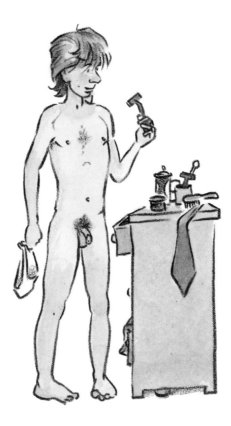

Boys: Puberty Changes

- Testicles gradually grow larger and fuller.
- Penis gradually grows larger and longer.
- Body sweats more.
- Skin and hair become more oily.
- Body has a sudden growth spurt.
- Body gains weight and grows taller.
- Arms and legs grow longer.
- Hands and feet grow larger.
- Bones in the face grow, and the face looks less childlike.
- Soft, darkish hair grows around the base of the penis and later becomes curly, thick, and coarse.
- Hair grows under the arms.
- Shoulders and chest grow bigger.
- Bigger muscles develop.
- Scrotum turns a darker color.
- Hair grows on the face, first the mustache, then the beard and sideburns.
- Hair grows on the chest.

PUBERTY FACT: Sometimes the area around a boy's nipples may feel sore and may even swell. This is caused by the hormones that are released during puberty. The soreness and swelling go away after a few months.

- The larynx, or as it is commonly called, the voice box, grows bigger.
- The voice cracks and then becomes deeper.
- The Adam's apple may begin to show more.

PUBERTY FACT: When a boy's voice begins to change, one second it can sound high, one second low, and the next high again, causing a cracking-squeaky sound. But after a while, a boy's voice begins to sound deeper and lower, because the larynx and vocal chords have grown. As the larynx grows bigger, it may push the Adam's apple forward, causing it to show more.

- Sperm begin to be produced.
- Ejaculations—including wet dreams—begin to occur.

PUBERTY FACT: Once a male can make sperm, if he has intercourse and if the female's ovaries have started to release eggs, she can become pregnant.

At this age, kids' bodies change more dramatically and rapidly than at any other time in their lives—except for the very first year of life.

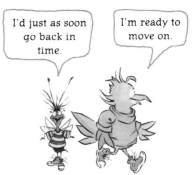

I'd just as soon go back in time.

I'm ready to move on.

14
More Changes
Taking Care of Your Body

Many of the physical changes that take place during puberty cause kids' bodies to work in many new ways. This means that kids have to learn some new ways to take care of their bodies.

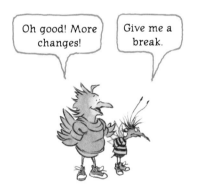

Girls and boys grow more hair during puberty. They grow hair under their arms. The hair on their arms and legs grows thicker and longer—especially boys' hair.

Hair called pubic hair also grows—for a girl around her vulva, and for a boy around the base of his penis—directly in front of a bone called the pubic bone.

The amount of hair that grows on boys' faces, chests, arms, and legs during puberty varies greatly, from hardly any to a lot.

Some boys and girls start shaving during puberty. For most, shaving is a choice. Some females choose to shave the hair that grows under their arms and on their legs, and some don't. Some males choose to shave their beards and mustaches, and some don't. However, some religious groups require that their boys and men not use a razor or scissors to cut their hair.

During puberty, a person's sweat glands produce more sweat than before. Both boys and girls start to sweat under their arms and develop a new kind of body odor, sometimes from under their arms, sometimes from their feet, and sometimes from all over their bodies.

That's one of the reasons kids going through puberty take a lot of baths or showers and wash their bodies and hair a lot. This new kind of sweating is often one of the first signs that puberty is starting. Washing with soap and using a deodorant can help get rid of most strong body odors.

Some kids sweat a lot. Some kids sweat a little. It is likely that you will sweat about the same amount as your father or mother did while he or she was going through puberty.

Some kids' hair becomes oily during puberty. Often some oiliness also begins to appear on kids' noses and foreheads.

During puberty, most boys

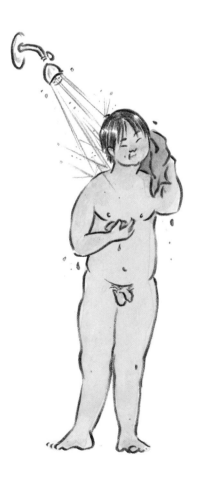

and girls develop pimples on their faces—mostly on their noses and foreheads. Sometimes, kids develop pimples on their backs and chests. Many kids call pimples "zits."

Although careful washing with soap and water is a good way to care for the skin, sometimes it is not enough. Creams and medicines can help control pimples. Some creams and medicines can be purchased directly at a drugstore without a doctor's written prescription; others need to be prescribed by a doctor and then purchased from a pharmacist.

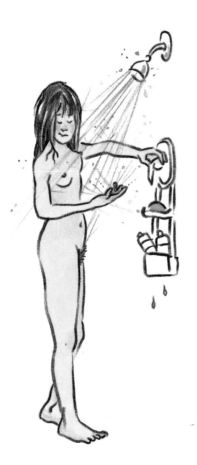

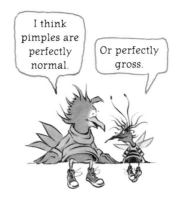

Though it's true that no one likes having pimples, having them is perfectly normal. Kids develop pimples and/or oily hair and sweat more during puberty because their oil and sweat glands are more active than ever before.

Puberty is the time when many girls, if they choose to, start to wear bras. *Bra* is short for the word *brassiere*. A girl often goes with her mother, grandmother, older sister, aunt, or a friend to buy her first bra.

It is not necessary to wear a bra to keep breasts healthy. Girls and women who wear bras do so because they feel more comfortable wearing them. Some wear a bra only when they are exercising or playing a sport. Others wear one all the time, except when sleeping. Still others never wear a bra at all. No matter what size breasts a girl or woman has, she can buy a bra that fits her. Bras are made with different size cups in order to support various breast sizes.

Many boys and men wear jockstraps when playing sports. A jockstrap fits over the testicles and penis, keeping them in place and protecting them from bruises or injuries. When playing some contact sports such as football or hockey or lacrosse, a male can slip a plastic cup, called an athletic cup, into the front of his jockstrap to provide even more protection for his testicles and penis. Athletic cups also come in various sizes.

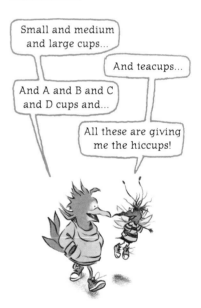

Kids' bodies change in so many ways during puberty that taking care of them can at times be a chore. However, eating healthy foods, exercising and keeping fit, keeping clean, and getting enough sleep can help a boy or girl feel healthy and good about all the growing and changing that go on.

15
Back and Forth, Up and Down
New and Changing Feelings

The many changes that take place in kids' bodies during puberty are often accompanied by new and strong feelings about how their bodies look, feel, and act—and by new and strong feelings about growing up and sex.

Many kids find these changes exciting and feel great about their bodies. And just as many find these changes overwhelming and feel shy or embarrassed about their changing bodies. Most kids, at one time or another during puberty, feel confused, uncomfortable, and even scared by these big and sometimes rapid changes.

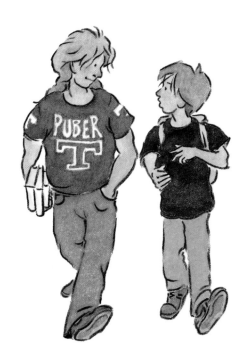

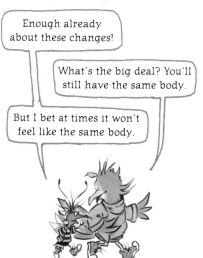

Enough already about these changes!

What's the big deal? You'll still have the same body.

But I bet at times it won't feel like the same body.

Kids often wonder about the size of individual body parts. The truth is—whether small, medium, or large—the size of a person's body parts has nothing to do with how well they work.

It is also true that different kids' bodies develop in different ways. Some girls develop small breasts, others develop medium-sized breasts, and still others develop large breasts. Some boys develop small penises, others develop medium-sized penises, and still other develop large penises. Breasts and penises come in all sorts of sizes.

A girl who develops small breasts may resemble her mother, grandmother, or another female relative. And a boy who develops little body hair may resemble his father, grandfather, or another male relative. The size of any part of a person's body is mostly inherited from a person's family.

The age when a boy or girl begins puberty is often the same as it was for a close family member of the same sex. You might

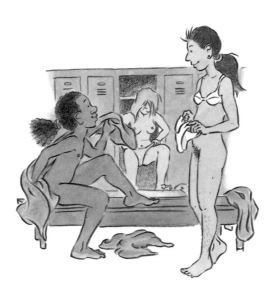

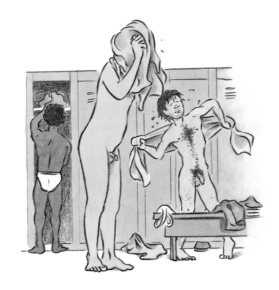

want to ask your mother, father, or other members of your family what puberty was like for them and when they began to go through it. You might find some clues about how you may develop.

Kids often wonder whether it matters if their bodies go through puberty slow or fast, early or late, or first or last. When your body changes, or how fast or slowly your body changes, has nothing to do with how your body will look and perform.

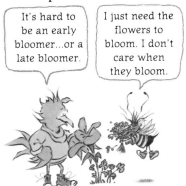

> It's hard to be an early bloomer...or a late bloomer.

> I just need the flowers to bloom. I don't care when they bloom.

Even so, among one's friends or in one's class, it can be hard to be the first or last girl who menstruates, or the first or last boy whose voice changes; or the first or last girl to wear a bra, or the first or last boy to shave; or the shortest kid one year and the tallest the next year.

Unfortunately, kids tease other kids about the ways their bodies look and grow during puberty. A kid's arms, hands, legs, and feet may grow longer and bigger before the rest of his or her body catches up. Or a boy's voice may crack right in the middle of a sentence. Or a girl may develop a large pimple on her forehead just before going to a party. Often these are the kinds of things kids are teased about as they go through puberty.

Many kids worry about their friendships during puberty— probably because puberty is a time when some kids start to have boyfriends or girlfriends. One of your friends, even your best friend, may begin to be interested in and sexually attracted to other kids, whereas you are not the least bit interested. One of your friends may start to have a boyfriend or girlfriend. Or you may have a boyfriend or girlfriend when your best friend doesn't.

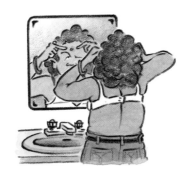

Sometimes kids feel upset or jealous when a friend has a boyfriend or a girlfriend and starts spending time with that person. Although many old friendships stay strong during puberty, some friendships change. Boyfriends and girlfriends are another thing kids are teased about during puberty.

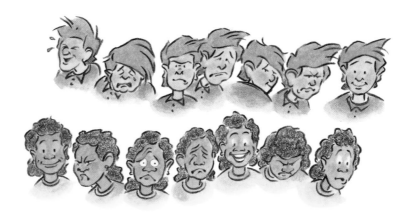

With all the different things that happen to their bodies during puberty, it's no wonder both boys and girls have so many different feelings. Kids can often feel moody or crabby or even teary and cry more than usual. And their moods can change quickly. A boy or girl may be laughing at one moment and feel like crying the next.

These different feelings often swing back and forth and up and down, like a yo-yo. The increased activity of the sex hormones is one of many factors that causes kids to have mood swings as well as new and strong feelings during puberty.

As kids' bodies change into grown-up bodies, kids are not always sure that they are ready to be grown-up. Sometimes they want to be treated as kids. Other times they want to be treated as adults.

Changing from a kid to an adult has its difficult moments. But sooner or later, kids get used to, become comfortable with, and feel good about their more grown-up bodies.

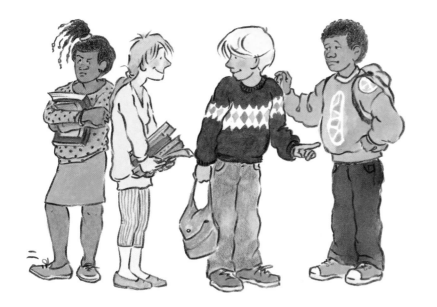

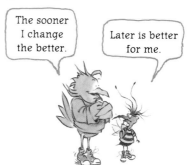

The sooner I change the better.

Later is better for me.

16
Perfectly Normal
Masturbation

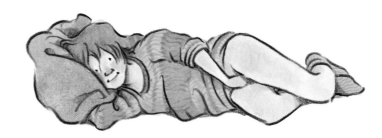

During puberty, when the sex hormones cause boys' and girls' sex organs to become more active, many kids begin to have even more pleasurable and excited feelings about their own bodies—and they may also be more attracted to and interested in other people's bodies.

These feelings are often called sexual feelings or "feeling sexy." Even though they are hard to describe, they are normal feelings. They happen at different times and in different ways for different kids.

Boys and girls, teenagers, and grown-ups too, experience sexy feelings when they masturbate. Masturbation is touching or rubbing any of your body's sex organs for pleasure—because it feels good. One everyday term for masturbating is "playing with yourself."

Some people think that masturbation is wrong or harmful. And some religions call masturbation a sin. But masturbating cannot hurt you. Many people masturbate. Many don't. Whether you masturbate or not is your choice. Masturbating is perfectly normal.

When people masturbate, they usually rub their sex organs with their hands or with something soft, like a pillow. A girl often rubs her clitoris; a boy often rubs his penis. Both the clitoris and the penis are sensitive to touch.

A person may have a warm, good, tingly, exciting feeling all through her or his body while masturbating. This feeling can become more and more intense

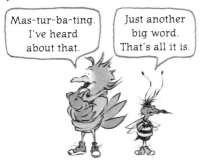

Mas-tur-ba-ting. I've heard about that.

Just another big word. That's all it is.

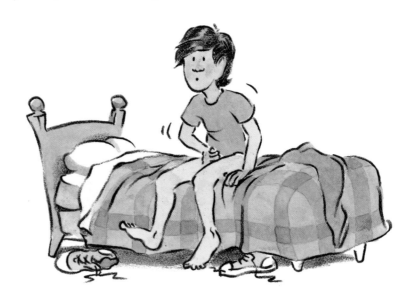

until it reaches a peak or climax. At that moment, a male may ejaculate; a female may feel strong, exciting sensations just in the area around her vulva or throughout her body. A female may also feel some wetness in her vagina.

For both females and males, this is called having an orgasm. Some people call it "coming." After having an orgasm, a person usually feels quite content and relaxed.

Usually, but not always, people have orgasms when they masturbate or when they have sexual intercourse. Both boys and girls may also have orgasms during a dream. People may have orgasms at some times and not at other times. Not everyone has orgasms.

Often when people masturbate, they daydream about someone or something happy or pleasurable or sexy. Some people become sexually excited without masturbating, just by looking at sexy pictures or by dreaming about or having fantasies about something pleasurable.

People of all ages masturbate—babies, kids, teenagers, grown-ups, and the elderly. Girls and boys often start to masturbate at puberty, but many start before.

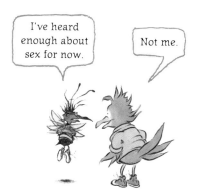

Part 4
Families and Babies

17
All Sorts of Families
Taking Care of Babies and Kids

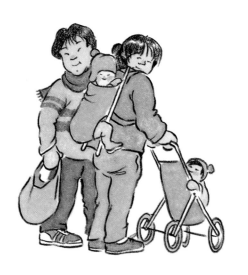

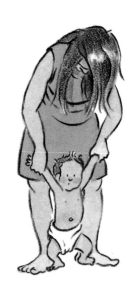

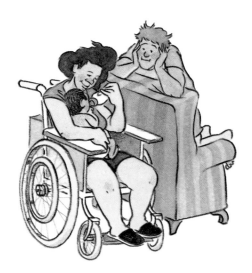

Babies and children grow up in all sorts of families. There are kids whose mother and father live together, or whose mother and father live apart, or who have only one parent, or whose parent or parents have adopted them, or who live with a parent and a step-parent, or who live with an aunt, an uncle, a grandmother, a grandfather, or other relative, or who have gay or lesbian parents, or who have foster parents.

Grandparents and cousins and uncles and aunts are also

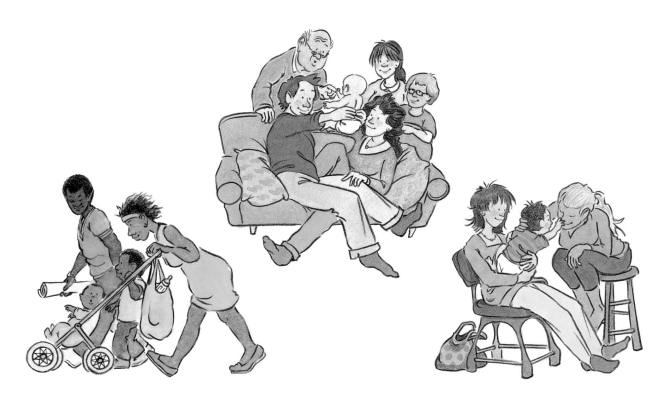

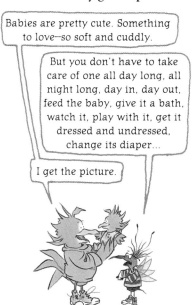

part of a person's family. And some people feel that their good friends are part of their families too. Most kids are loved and taken care of by family members and family friends.

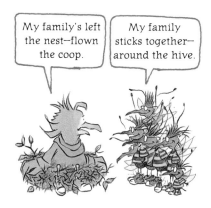

My family's left the nest—flown the coop.

My family sticks together—around the hive.

Bringing a baby into this world is an important and exciting event. Becoming a parent is one of the biggest changes that can happen to a person. It brings with it all sorts of new and different responsibilities.

These responsibilities include taking good care of oneself as well as of one's baby and family. That's why the decision about when to start a family is so important. Although it is physically possible for a girl and a boy to make a baby once the girl has started to menstruate (and in rare instances, even before) and once the boy has begun to produce sperm, it makes good sense for people to wait until they are ready and old enough to take on such big responsibilities.

Having a baby when a person is too young can be difficult. There are lots of reasons for this.

Babies of kids and young teen-agers are often born weighing too little even after a full nine months in the uterus. Babies who weigh too little are more likely to have health problems at birth and as they grow up.

Babies are pretty cute. Something to love—so soft and cuddly.

But you don't have to take care of one all day long, all night long, day in, day out, feed the baby, give it a bath, watch it, play with it, get it dressed and undressed, change its diaper...

I get the picture.

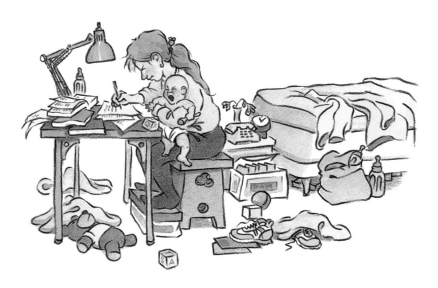

Parents often find it hard to care for a baby, especially if they are still kids or young teenagers. Kids or young teenagers who have a baby often lose the freedom to do what they want to do. It's hard to go out with friends or to get schoolwork done when a baby is around. Babies need a lot of attention, day in, day out, every day, every night.

Teenagers who have babies often have to drop out of school because they need to work. It costs a lot of money to buy food, clothes, toys, and medicine for a baby. It's often hard for teenagers to get a job to pay for these things. And it costs a lot of money to pay someone else to take care of a baby while they go to school or to work.

Babies are very special and most mothers and fathers love their babies a lot. But it's usually easier and healthier for kids and teenagers to wait until they are older to have a baby. It gives the baby and the parents a better chance to have a healthy start together.

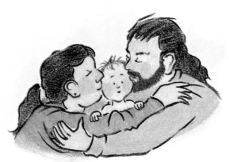

18
Instructions from Mom and Dad
The Cell: Genes and Chromosomes

All living creatures start out as a single cell. When two sex cells—an egg and a sperm—unite into a single cell, they carry all the information required to make a new baby—a new human being. This information is stored in more than one hundred thousand genes in the center of the cell.

Some scientists describe a person's genes as little packages of instructions. Your packages of instructions, that is, your genes, helped to decide all sorts of things about you—whether you are male or female, the color of your eyes, the shape of your ears, the type and color of your hair, and the color of your skin.

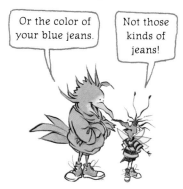

Or the color of your blue jeans.

Not those kinds of jeans!

Your genes were passed on to you from both your parents, and through them from their parents, and through them from earlier generations on both sides of your family. And many of your genes will be passed on to your children and grandchildren.

Genes are made of DNA—a short name for a chemical called deoxyribonucleic acid. Genes are carried on long, threadlike strings of DNA called chromosomes. A gene is a tiny part of a chromosome. A chromosome is the part of each cell that carries a person's genes. You might picture a chromosome as a string of beads, with each bead as a gene.

A chromosome

Every cell in the human body has forty-six chromosomes. But each egg cell and each sperm cell carries only twenty-three chromosomes. If an egg and a sperm unite, the combined single cell has a grand total of forty-six chromosomes.

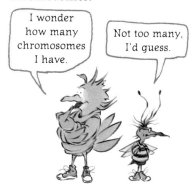

I wonder how many chromosomes I have.

Not too many, I'd guess.

That means half your chromosomes, as well as half your DNA, comes from your mother and the other half comes from your father. You received a combination of genes from both of them. That's why, while you are not an exact copy of either one of your parents, you probably do resemble each of them in some ways.

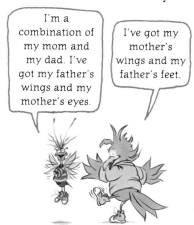

I'm a combination of my mom and my dad. I've got my father's wings and my mother's eyes.

I've got my mother's wings and my father's feet.

If two eggs leave the ovaries at the same time, and if each egg is fertilized by a separate sperm, fraternal, or nonidentical, twins

begin. Since fraternal twins do not have the same genes, they do not look exactly like each other and can be the same sex or the opposite sex.

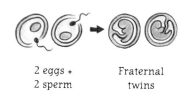

2 eggs + 2 sperm

Fraternal twins

Identical twins begin if a single egg splits into two after it has been fertilized. Since identical twins have the same genes, they are always the same sex and look almost exactly like each other.

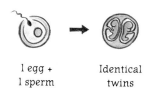

1 egg + 1 sperm

Identical twins

When two or more babies are born at the same birth—twins, triplets, and so on—it is called a multiple birth.

Unless you are an identical twin, you are not an exact genetic copy of your brother or sister, because a different sperm and egg unite to form every new baby. Each sperm and each egg carries a different combination of genes. That's why you can look somewhat different or very different from your sister or brother.

Scientists have discovered that a person's gender—female or male—is determined the moment the egg and sperm unite.

Among the twenty-three chromosomes in each egg cell and each sperm cell is one sex chromosome. There are two kinds of sex chromosomes—either an X or a Y. All eggs carry an X chromosome and all sperm carry either an X or a Y chromosome. If an egg is fertilized by a sperm with a Y chromosome, the united single cell will develop into a baby boy—XY. And if an egg is fertilized by a sperm with an X chromosome, the united single cell will develop into a baby girl—XX.

Whether you are male or female was determined by which chromosome—an X or a Y—was in the sperm from your father that fertilized your mother's egg.

The genes inside your body carry lots of information about you and determine many things—but not everything—about you.

Where you are brought up and how you are brought up, including the kind of food you eat and the kind of exercise you get, as well as the people who are around you and the events that occur as you grow up, also help to shape many things about you. That's why no two people in the world—even identical twins—are exactly alike. Each of us is unique.

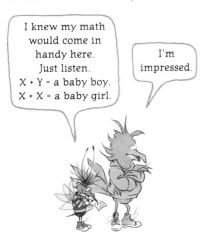

I knew my math would come in handy here. Just listen. X + Y = a baby boy. X + X = a baby girl.

I'm impressed.

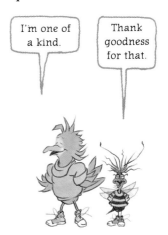

I'm one of a kind.

Thank goodness for that.

19

A Kind of Sharing
Cuddling, Kissing, Touching, and Sexual Intercourse

Sexual intercourse, or as it is often called, "making love," is a kind of sharing between two people. The very beginnings of a new human being—a baby—can form, immediately after sexual intercourse, if a sperm cell joins with an egg cell.

Touching, caressing, kissing, and hugging—often called "making out" or "petting"—are other kinds of sharing that can make two people feel very close and loving and excited about one another. People can and do become sexually excited without having sexual intercourse. Choosing to wait to have sexual

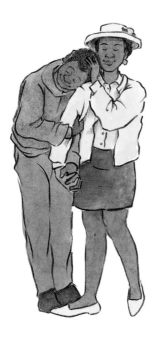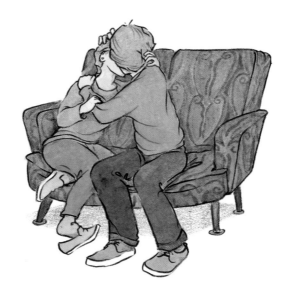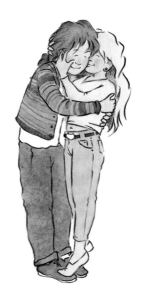

intercourse until one is older or feels more responsible is called postponement. Choosing not to have sexual intercourse is called abstinence.

When two people feel they are too young to have sexual intercourse, do not know each other well enough, or do not want to have sexual intercourse for any other reason, they may decide just to hold hands, cuddle, dance, kiss, or make out.

Sharing between two people who care about each other always means having respect for each other's feelings and wishes, including respecting each other's

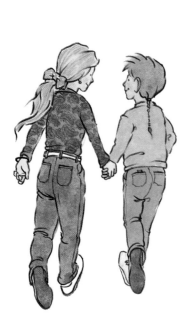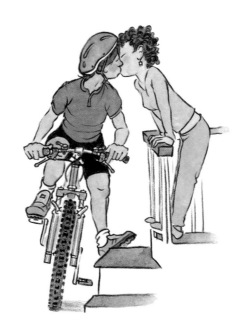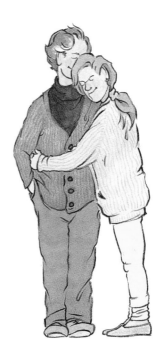

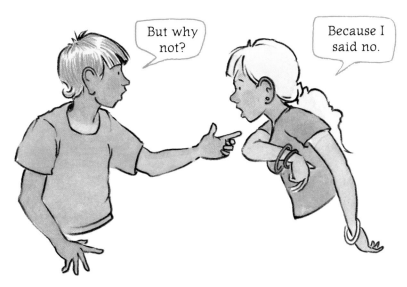

But why not?

Because I said no.

right to say no to any kind of sexual activity—any time and for any reason.

Sexual intercourse usually begins with two people touching, caressing, kissing, and hugging each other.

After a bit, the female's vagina becomes moist and slippery, her clitoris becomes hard, and the male's penis becomes erect, stiff, and larger. Sometimes a bit of clear fluid that may contain a few sperm comes out of the tip of the penis and makes it wet. The female and male begin to feel excited about each other.

All this sounds exciting.

It sounds gross and messy. I don't want to hear any more about it.

It is now possible for the male's erect penis to go inside the female's vagina, which stretches in a way that fits around the penis. The moisture from the vagina makes it easier for the penis to go in.

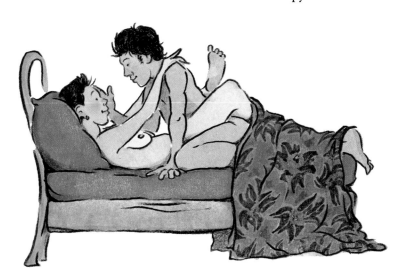

During sexual intercourse, as the male and female move back and forth in rhythm, the movement of the penis inside the vagina soon feels very good. The female and male may hug and kiss and touch each other even more as all of this is going on and feel more and more excited.

When these feelings come to a climax, semen is ejaculated from the penis and spurts into the vagina, and the muscles in the vagina and uterus tighten and finally relax. A small amount of fluid may come out of the vagina. This is called "having an orgasm."

A female and male may have orgasms at different times. And sometimes one person has an orgasm and the other doesn't. After an orgasm, most people feel relaxed, content, and sometimes even sleepy.

Every time a couple has sexual intercourse it can result in a baby—unless the female is already pregnant.

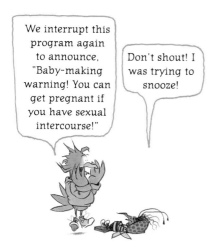

People have a lot of mistaken ideas about how a girl or woman who has had sexual intercourse can and cannot become pregnant. It's important to know that a girl or woman can become pregnant even if she is standing up during sexual intercourse; even if it is the very first time she has had sexual intercourse; even if she has had sexual intercourse only once; even if she thinks or feels she is menstruating; even if she does not have an orgasm.

A girl or woman can also become pregnant even if the boy or man pulls out before he ejaculates. If sperm are ejaculated close to the opening of the vagina —or even if just a few sperm spurt out before ejaculation—it is possible for them to swim up the vagina and join with an egg.

This can also happen even when a female and a male do not have sexual intercourse, if sperm are ejaculated close to the opening to the vagina.

However, if a couple decides to have sexual intercourse, there are ways—called birth control—that can help protect them from having a baby.

And a couple can help protect each other from getting infections that are spread by sexual contact if they use a condom correctly and every time they have sex. This is one way of practicing "safer sex."

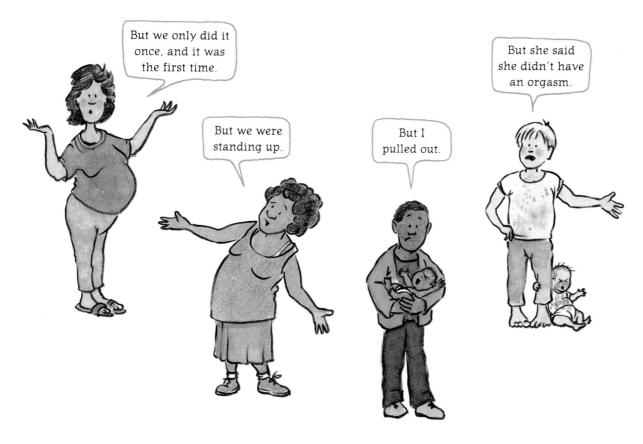

20
Before Birth
Pregnancy

The word *pregnant* comes from two Latin words: *prae*, which means before, and *gnas*, which means birth.

Pregnancy is the period of time before birth during which a fertilized egg plants itself inside the lining of the uterus, grows inside the uterus, and eventually develops into a baby. The union of a sperm and an egg is called conception or fertilization.

Scientists have discovered exactly how a pregnancy begins by observing how sperm travel, meet, and finally unite with an egg.

Living sperm are great travelers, and it is wonderful to watch them move under a microscope. You can actually see their tails move rapidly back and forth.

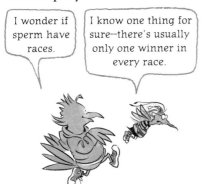

I wonder if sperm have races.

I know one thing for sure—there's usually only one winner in every race.

They look like tadpoles swimming and travel like a school of fish—in large groups of about five hundred million.

When sperm are ejaculated in the female's vagina during sexual intercourse, they swim up the vagina, through the cervix, into the uterus, and into the Fallopian tubes. If an egg has been released and swept into one of the Fallopian tubes, a sperm can unite with it and fertilize it—and the female can become pregnant.

Only about two hundred sperm out of the five hundred million in an ejaculation get close to the egg.

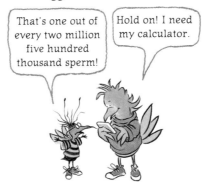

That's one out of every two million five hundred thousand sperm!

Hold on! I need my calculator.

Scientists have shown that a chemical in the fluid around the egg actually attracts certain sperm, telling them that the egg

is ready, and lets only one sperm out of those two hundred or so break into the egg cell. After that sperm enters the egg, none of the others can get in, and fertilization takes place.

Once an egg cell unites with a sperm cell, it becomes a single cell—the first cell of a baby. A fertilized egg cell is called a zygote from conception and for the next several days as it travels to the uterus; an embryo during the next two months as it develops in the uterus; and a fetus throughout the rest of the pregnancy—until a baby is born. Some people call the fetus a "developing baby."

The fertilized egg cell takes about five days to travel through the Fallopian tube and into the uterus, dividing again and again. Inside the uterus, it plants itself in the uterus's lining, where it will grow and develop into a baby. The uterus is also called "the womb."

While in the uterus, a fertilized egg cell continues to divide billions and billions of times to

THE FURTHER ADVENTURES OF THE EGG AND SPERM: *Pregnancy*

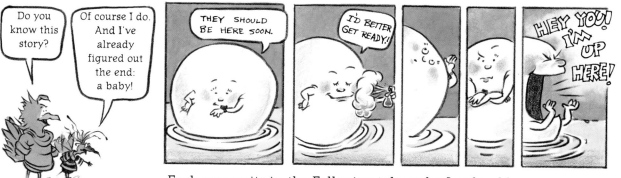

Each egg waits in the Fallopian tube to be fertilized by a sperm.

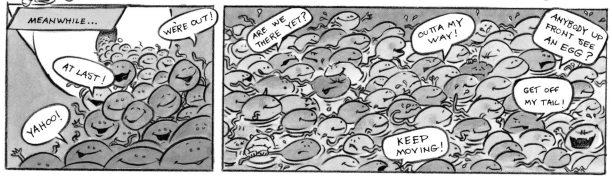

Sperm leave the penis, swim up the vagina, through the uterus,

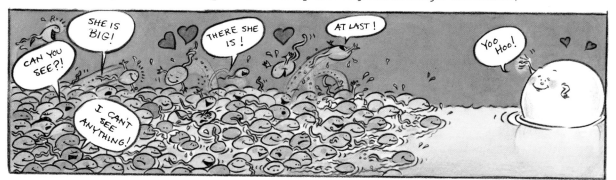

and into a Fallopian tube where an egg may be waiting to unite with a sperm.

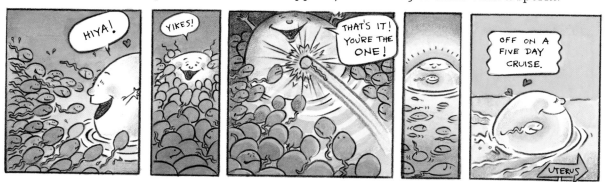

If one sperm enters the egg, they become one cell and pregnancy can begin.

From Zygote to Baby — 9 Months

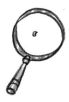 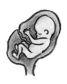 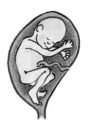 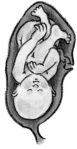

Zygote—*day 1*   Embryo—*month 1*   Fetus—*month 3*   Fetus—*month 6*   Baby about to be born—*month 9*

make billions and billions of new cells. Eventually, over nine months, these cells become a whole new person—a baby.

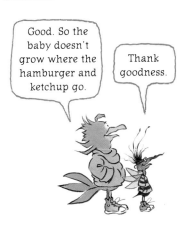

I wonder how long it takes a bee cell to grow into a bee.

21 days.

It takes a bird cell, depending on its cell size, anywhere from 10 to 74 days.

With the size of your birdbrain...I'd say 10 days.

In the uterus, a sac filled with a watery fluid forms around the developing baby and protects it against pokes, bumps, and jolts. The sac is called the amniotic sac or the "bag of waters," and the fluid is called amniotic fluid. This fluid is warm and keeps the

developing baby warm as it floats.

A lot of kids and even some grown-ups think that the developing baby grows in the mother's stomach. It does not grow in the stomach.

Good. So the baby doesn't grow where the hamburger and ketchup go.

Thank goodness.

It grows in the uterus. As the developing baby grows bigger, the uterus also grows bigger.

As the embryo fastens itself to the inside of the uterus, a special organ called the placenta forms inside the uterus. During pregnancy, the placenta supplies the

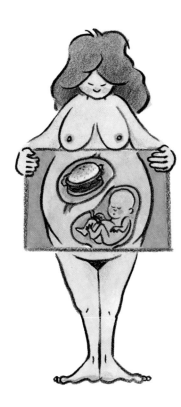

embryo and—later on—the fetus with oxygen from the air the mother breathes and nutrients from the food she eats.

Nutrients are made up of vitamins, proteins, fats, sugars, carbohydrates, and water— all the things a fetus needs in order to grow into a healthy baby.

The umbilical cord—a soft, bendable tube—connects the placenta to the fetus at the umbilicus. The word *umbilicus* means navel, and *navel* is another word for "belly button."

Oxygen and nutrients travel from the placenta to the fetus in the blood that flows through the umbilical cord. The oxygen and nutrients, as well as other substances from the mother, pass from her blood into the fetus's blood.

The fetus's waste—liquids and solids that are left over from the nutrients not used by the fetus—travel back through the umbilical cord to the placenta and pass into the mother's blood. The fetus's

waste leaves the mother's body along with the mother's waste.

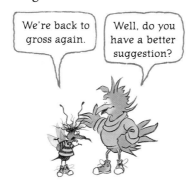

We're back to gross again.

Well, do you have a better suggestion?

Medicines, drugs, and alcohol can also pass into the fetus's blood from the mother's blood. That's why a pregnant female should be very careful about what she eats, drinks, and puts into her body. If she needs to take a prescription drug, she should check with her doctor or nurse to make sure the

drug will not hurt the fetus.

If a female has abused drugs, consumed alcohol, smoked cigarettes, not eaten healthy foods, or had certain kinds of infections while pregnant, her baby could be born with or develop serious health problems. It could have difficulty eating and breathing and growing properly. And if a pregnant mother has been addicted to drugs, her baby may be born addicted to drugs.

However, if a pregnant mother takes good care of herself—has regular checkups with a nurse or doctor, eats healthy food, and gets enough exercise and sleep—her baby will have the best chance to be born healthy.

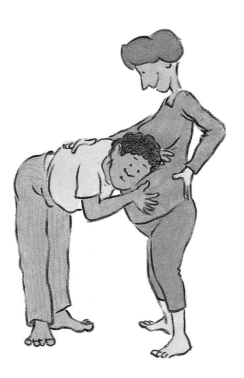

21
What a Trip!
Birth

The birth of a baby is almost always a healthy and joyful event. A pregnant woman knows that her baby is ready to be born when she can feel the muscles of her uterus tighten and squeeze and then relax, over and over, many times in a row.

The woman's muscles are actually beginning to push the baby out of her uterus. All this tightening and squeezing and pushing is called labor. *Labor* is another word for *work*.

When labor starts, the pregnant woman usually goes to a hospital unless she has arranged to have the birth at home with a doctor or a midwife and a nurse. A midwife—a person who has been specially trained to help a woman deliver a baby—is not a doctor but may be a nurse. Fathers, and sometimes other family members and friends, can also help the mother during labor and birth. Labor can be as short as an hour or longer than a whole day.

After labor has started, and occasionally before, the amniotic sac—the bag of waters—breaks, and fluid begins to leak out. This can be another sign that the baby is ready to be born.

During the birth, the baby travels out of the uterus, through the cervix, which has opened and widened during labor, and into the vagina. The vagina stretches as the baby travels through it and out of the mother's body.

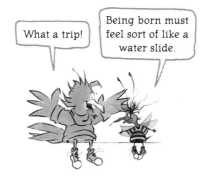

The vagina is often called the "birth canal," because *canal* is another word for *passageway*.

In most births, the baby's head pushes out of the vagina first. Any fluid in its mouth or nose is carefully taken out so the baby can breathe on its own. Then the rest of its body comes out. Usually the doctor, midwife, or father gently holds the new-born baby as it comes out. This is called a vaginal birth.

Some babies need to be gently pulled out by tongs, called forceps. This is called a forceps birth. And some babies come out of the uterus and vagina feet first. This is called a breech birth.

Other babies are too big to travel safely through the vagina. Or they are in positions that make it difficult for them to travel out of the uterus and through the vagina on their own.

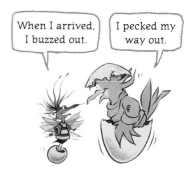

If the baby is too big or in an awkward position, the doctor makes a side-to-side cut through the mother's skin—after it has been made numb with a special medicine—into the mother's uterus and lifts the baby and the placenta out. Then the doctor

WHAT A TRIP!: *Birth*

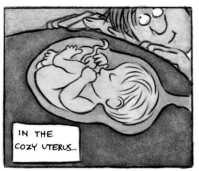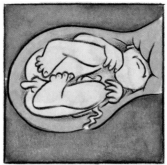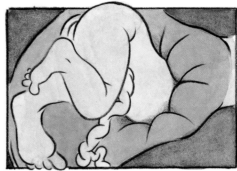

When it's time to be born, the mother's muscles squeeze and push the baby out

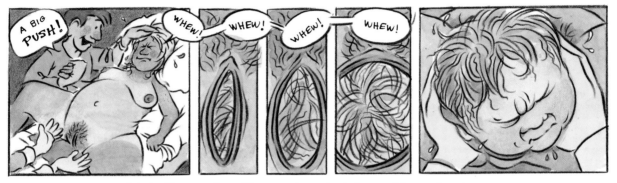

and into the vagina. The vagina stretches wide and out comes

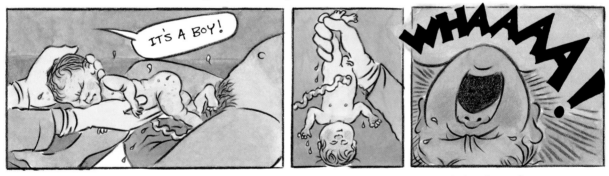

the baby, who is still connected to the mother by the umbilical cord,

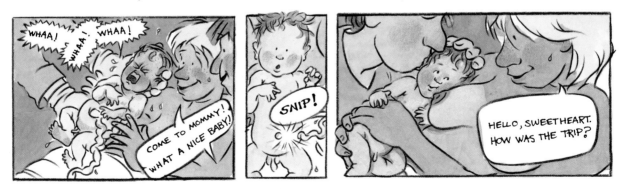

which is cut. And right away, the new baby is cuddled and held.

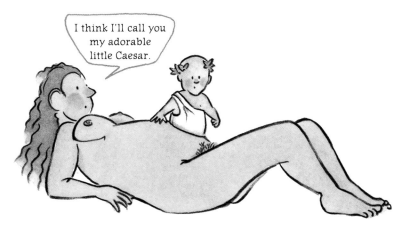

I think I'll call you my adorable little Caesar.

feelings of love and awe. These fond and loving feelings between parents and their child often begin at birth, but they can also begin in the weeks after birth.

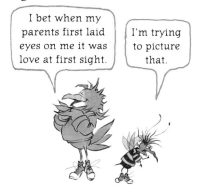

I bet when my parents first laid eyes on me it was love at first sight.

I'm trying to picture that.

cuts the umbilical cord and sews up the mother's cut, which heals in a few weeks' time.

This is called a cesarean birth, or "c-section," and is another healthy way for a baby to be born. It is believed that the term *cesarean* dates back to the time of Julius Caesar, the great Roman leader, general, and politician, who may have been born this way around 100 B.C.—more than two thousand years ago.

A forceps birth, a breech birth, and a cesarean birth are perfectly normal ways for a baby to be born. No matter which way a baby is born, right after birth it takes its first breath and lets out its first cry. This allows its lungs to open up and begin to work on their own. The moment of birth is so exciting!

Even though the baby is still attached to the placenta by the umbilical cord, it does not need the placenta anymore. The doctor or midwife places a clamp on the baby's umbilical cord and

then cuts the cord about an inch from the baby's navel. Since there are no nerve endings in the umbilical cord, neither the baby nor the mother can feel the cut.

A few days later, the clamped piece of umbilical cord dries out and falls off painlessly. The place where it was attached becomes a person's navel, or belly button.

After the cord has been cut, the muscles of the uterus give a few more squeezes and pushes, and the placenta and amniotic sac slide out. Because they leave the mother's body after the baby has been born, they are called the afterbirth.

As soon as possible, the newborn baby is gently dried off, wrapped in a blanket, and given to the mother or father to cuddle and hold.

When parents are first given their newborn baby to hold and can feel the baby's skin against their skin and can feel the baby breathe, they have—more often than not—new and special

A newborn baby is usually weighed and measured and given some eye drops to prevent infection a few minutes after it is born.

The birth of a baby is a fascinating event. At birth, a baby can see, hear, cry, suck, grab, feel, and smell. And it can eat by sucking from its mother's breast or from a bottle. A newborn baby can do an amazing number of things.

If a boy baby is to be circumcised, that is, if the foreskin of his penis is to be removed, either by a doctor or a person who learned to perform circumcision as part of a religious ceremony, it is usually done a few days after birth. It takes only a few minutes to perform a circumcision.

Some circumcisions are performed for religious reasons. Baby boys who are born into the

Jewish or Muslim faith are usually circumcised as part of a religious ceremony.

Other circumcisions are performed for health reasons—to make it easier to keep the tip of the boy's penis clean. However, an uncircumcised penis can be kept clean by pulling back the foreskin and gently washing the tip. Most doctors feel that the penis can be kept clean whether it is circumcised or not.

Some parents like the idea of having their son look like his father, and sometimes that's how they make the decision about whether their baby boy is going to be circumcised.

Babies are born in many different ways. Some babies are born early, before they have spent a full nine months in the uterus. This is called a premature birth. A baby who is born early is called a premature baby or a "preemie."

A baby who is born only two or three weeks early has grown big enough to have a healthy start in life and can usually go home with its parents after one or two days in the hospital. But if a baby is born a month or more early, living outside the uterus can be hard. The baby's lungs may not be fully developed, making it difficult for the baby to breathe. The baby may not be able to suck or swallow easily, making it difficult for the baby to eat. And the baby may have trouble staying warm.

A baby who is born a month or more early usually has to stay in the hospital until he or she is healthy enough to go home. In the hospital, the baby stays in a specially equipped crib called an incubator, which keeps the baby warm and provides oxygen—just as the mother's uterus did for the fetus—while it continues to grow. While the baby is in the incubator, the baby's parents, the doctors, and the nurses feed and take care of the baby.

When the baby has grown big

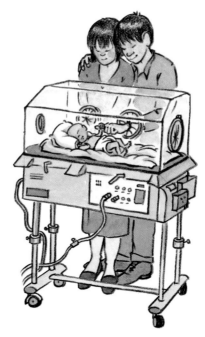

enough and is close to being as healthy as a baby who has spent a full nine months growing in the uterus, and can eat well and keep warm, its parents can take their baby home.

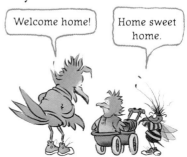

Welcome home!

Home sweet home.

22
Other Arrivals
More Ways to Have a Baby and Family

Sometimes people want to have a baby but cannot have one because their egg and sperm are not able to unite. Fortunately, there are ways other than sexual intercourse to have a baby.

There can be many different reasons why an egg cell and a sperm cell are not able to unite, such as the female's ovaries are not able to release an egg each month, an egg is not able to travel through the Fallopian tubes, too few sperm are able to travel to the egg, the male's sperm are too weak to travel to the egg.

However, with the help of a doctor, a female's egg can be fertilized by a male's sperm and a pregnancy can begin.

An egg can be taken out of one of the ovaries by a doctor and put into a small glass dish filled with fluid along with sperm that have been ejaculated. After the egg has been fertilized by one of the sperm in the dish, the egg is returned to the uterus, and a pregnancy can begin. This method of starting a pregnancy is called in vitro fertilization.

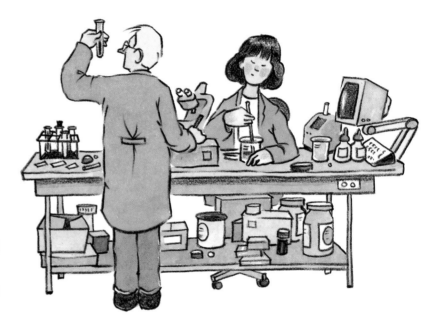

In vitro are the Latin words for *in a glass.*

When there are not enough sperm, or not enough sperm strong enough to swim to the egg, a doctor can place the male's ejaculated sperm in the female's vagina or uterus with a syringe. In the uterus, the sperm have a shorter distance to swim and a better chance of uniting with an egg in one of the Fallopian tubes.

Starting a pregnancy in this way is called artificial insemination—even though there is noth-

ing artificial about the egg and sperm or the uniting of the egg and sperm. *Inseminate* means *to put a seed in,* in other words, *to make pregnant.*

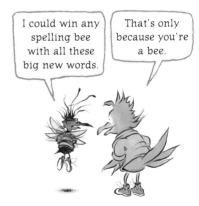

I could win any spelling bee with all these big new words.

That's only because you're a bee.

Sometimes, if a male becomes very sick, the medication he needs to become well may lessen the number of sperm that he is able to make. Before the male takes the medication, his ejaculated sperm can be placed in a sperm bank—a medical laboratory—to be frozen and stored for up to ten or fifteen years. It can be used later to conceive a baby by artificial insemination.

There are people who are not able to conceive a baby at all—by sexual intercourse, by in vitro fertilization, by artificial insemination, or by freezing sperm. However, they can start a family by adopting a baby or child.

Adoption means that a family will bring another family's baby or child into their family and raise that child as their very own. An adopted child becomes a member of his or her new family.

Many people choose to adopt children because they are not able to conceive a baby. Some people who can conceive a baby also choose to adopt children.

Adoption usually occurs when a parent or parents who are unable to take care of their newborn baby or child decide to have someone else care for, bring up, and love their baby or child.

Adoption is a legal act. This means that the child's birth parent or parents sign a paper in

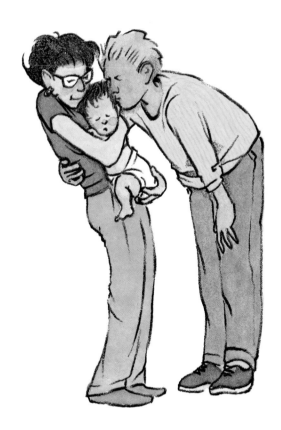

front of a lawyer or judge that says that they are giving their child forever to a parent or parents who want to and are able to take care of the child.

The new adoptive parent or parents agree to raise the child as their own. They too sign the

adoption paper in front of a lawyer or judge.

There are many ways to have a baby and create a family. But no matter how people have a child, caring for and loving one can be a wonderful and amazing experience.

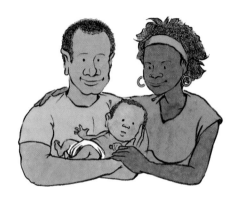

Part 5
Decisions

23
Planning Ahead
Postponement, Abstinence, and Birth Control

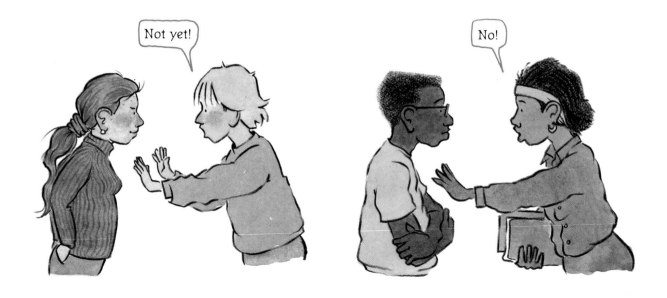

Not yet!

No!

Whether or not to have sexual intercourse is a decision each person has a right to make. But a person should always remember that sexual intercourse can result in pregnancy and having a baby.

Many young people choose to wait to have sexual intercourse until they feel they are either old enough or responsible enough. This is called postponement. *Postponement* means *to delay until a later time.*

However, the only sure way not to have an unwanted pregnancy is to not have sexual intercourse. This is called abstinence.

Abstinence means *to abstain, to keep from doing something you want to do.*

In addition to preventing the start of a pregnancy, postponement and abstinence can also help prevent a person from getting or passing on infections that are spread by sexual contact.

Many people who choose to postpone or abstain from sexual intercourse say that they can still have a close, loving, and sexy relationship with another person.

Sometimes, when people choose to have sexual intercourse, they have planned to have a baby. But other people may want to wait to have a baby or may not want to have a baby at all. That's why knowing how to prevent pregnancy is important.

Birth control and *contraception* are the two names given to the many ways of preventing a pregnancy.

Contra is the Latin word for *against*. *Ception* is part of the word *conception*, which means *beginning*. *Contraception* means *against beginning a pregnancy*.

There are many kinds of birth control, and some work better than others. A person must learn how to use them and must use them every time he or she has sexual intercourse in order for them to work. However, no method of birth control can be guaranteed to work 100 percent of the time.

Condoms, spermicide, and sponges are types of birth control that can be bought at a store, usually a drugstore. Often they are displayed on the counter—right next to the cash register.

That's why these kinds of birth control are called "over-the-counter contraceptives."

Condoms have been in use since the sixteenth century. A condom is a soft, very thin cover that fits over an erect penis. When a male ejaculates, semen is kept inside the condom and sperm are not able to unite with an egg. But sometimes semen can leak out. A condom works better to prevent pregnancy when used with a contraceptive foam, cream, or jelly—called a spermicide—that contains a chemical that can kill sperm.

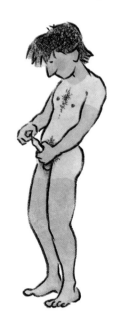

Putting on a condom

Using a condom during sexual intercourse, correctly and every time, can also help prevent the spread of infections—mild infections as well as life-threatening infections such as HIV and hepatitis B. This is a way of practicing safer sex. It's important for people to understand that any type of birth control method, when used by itself—*without* a condom—*cannot* prevent a person from getting an infection from or passing on an infection to another person.

Condoms are called "rubbers" because they are usually made out of a rubbery material called latex. A newer type of male condom, made out of a strong, fairly thin, rubbery material called polyurethane, is believed by scientists to be stronger than latex.

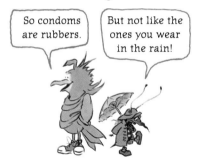

It is important for a person to use latex or polyurethane condoms, not lambskin, because they are less likely to leak or break.

A condom designed to fit inside the vagina, called the female condom, is also made out of polyurethane. This soft pouch-like condom is inserted into the vagina before sexual intercourse.

The chemical in spermicide—foams, creams, and jellies—and

in sponges can kill sperm, but sponges can also block sperm. These types of contraceptives are also inserted into the vagina before sexual intercourse. Spermicide and sponges should be used with condoms. When they are used alone, they are usually not able to kill, block, or catch every sperm or protect a person from getting or passing on an infection. It is important to use condoms with water-based lubricants made especially for sex and made with water, not oil, because oil can damage and break a latex condom.

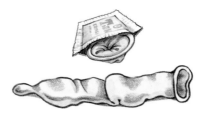

Condom

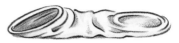

Female condom

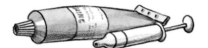

Spermicide

Sponge

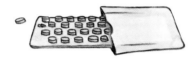

Birth control pills

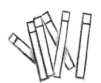

Norplant

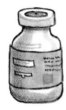

Depo Provera

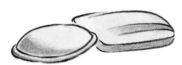

Diaphragm

Cervical cap

Intrauterine device

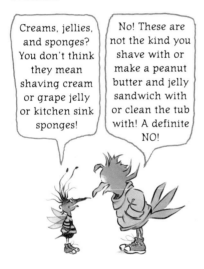

Creams, jellies, and sponges? You don't think they mean shaving cream or grape jelly or kitchen sink sponges!

No! These are not the kind you shave with or make a peanut butter and jelly sandwich with or clean the tub with! A definite NO!

Birth control pills, Norplant, Depo Provera, the diaphragm, the cervical cap, and the IUD are contraceptives that a female can obtain only after being examined by a trained health-care professional—a doctor, midwife, nurse practitioner, or physician's assistant—and obtaining a written prescription. The prescribed birth control method can then be obtained at a doctor's office or health clinic or purchased at a drugstore from a pharmacist.

Birth control pills, commonly called "the pill," contain artificial hormones that keep ovaries from releasing mature eggs. A female must remember to follow the

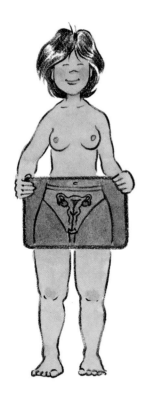

directions for taking a pill each day for this method of birth control to work.

Norplant is a birth control device that is placed in a female's upper arm just under her skin by a health-care professional. Its six tiny tubes slowly release an artificial hormone that keeps the ovaries from releasing mature eggs for up to five years.

Depo Provera is a birth control drug made of an artificial hormone that is injected in a female's upper arm once every three months and keeps the ovaries from releasing mature eggs.

The diaphragm and the cervical cap are small latex cups that fit inside the vagina and are placed against the cervix before sexual intercourse. Both can prevent sperm from entering the cervix and traveling to the Fallopian tubes. And both must be used with a spermicide.

An IUD, or intrauterine device, is a small plastic and copper device that is placed inside the uterus by a trained health-care professional and can prevent an egg from planting itself in the uterus's lining.

If a person makes the decision to have sexual intercourse, the most useful protection against pregnancy or infection is the correct use of birth control before or at the time of sexual intercourse.

However, if there is an emergency and a woman or girl has been raped—forced to have sex against her will—or if she has had unprotected sex for any reason, there is a pill—called the morning-after pill—that she can

Where They Fit

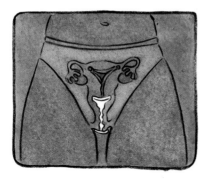

Female condom

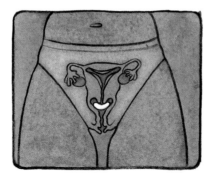

Sponge

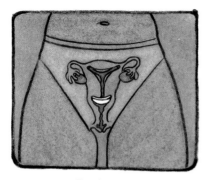

Diaphragm

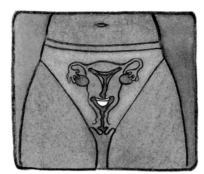

Cervical cap

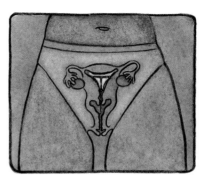

IUD

take to prevent the start of a pregnancy. It contains hormones that are thought to prevent fertilization or the planting of a fertilized egg in the lining of the uterus. This method of preventing a pregnancy must take place within seventy-two hours after sexual intercourse, under the supervision of a health-care professional. It should not be relied upon as a regular form of birth control.

Some methods of birth control, such as the rhythm method or the withdrawal method, are not considered effective.

When a male and female use the rhythm method, they try to figure out when the female's ovary has released an egg and then abstain from having sexual intercourse during that time. However, it is very difficult to know when an egg has been released, because the time can vary from month to month—especially for many teenage girls.

When a couple uses the withdrawal method, the male removes his penis from the female's vagina just before he ejaculates. This method does not work very well either because some semen often leaks out before ejaculation or because the male may fail to remove his penis before he ejaculates.

Sometimes when people decide not to have more children,

they may choose to have a simple operation called sterilization.

When a male has this operation—called a vasectomy—a small piece of the vas deferens is removed or tied off by a doctor. As a result, the semen that is ejaculated no longer carries any sperm.

When a female has this operation—called a tubal ligation—a small piece of each Fallopian tube is removed or tied off by a doctor so that an egg cannot get to the uterus and sperm cannot get to an egg.

Some religions and groups and some individuals believe that using any method of birth control is wrong. Others believe that using the rhythm method and withdrawal is fine, but that using over-the-counter and prescription birth control methods is wrong.

Still others think birth control is a fine and responsible way to prevent an unwanted pregnancy or delay having a baby. These people use birth control to help them plan a family.

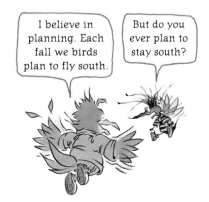

I believe in planning. Each fall we birds plan to fly south.

But do you ever plan to stay south?

A person's parents, doctor, nurse, and school nurse are good people to talk with about birth control, postponement, and abstinence. Neighborhood health clinics or family planning clinics are other good places to go for information.

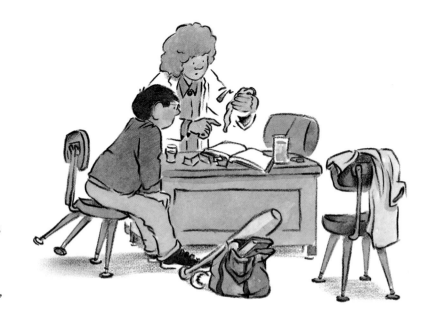

24
Laws and Rulings
Abortion

An abortion is a medical procedure performed for the purpose of ending a pregnancy. Some pregnant females choose to have abortions. People's feelings about having abortions are not always simple, however, and can range from relief to sadness, from worry to fear.

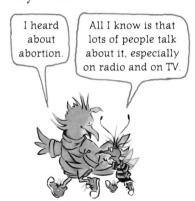

I heard about abortion.

All I know is that lots of people talk about it, especially on radio and on TV.

The word *abort* means *to stop* or *to end something at an early stage.* An abortion is usually performed in a clinic or a hospital by a doctor or other trained health-care professional and is a safe procedure when done early. The pregnancy is ended by removing the embryo or fetus from the uterus. The procedure itself takes about five minutes and is usually performed during the first three months of pregnancy, before most females even look pregnant.

There is an abortion pill called RU 486 that can end a pregnancy. It is used in some countries, but is not yet available in the United States, though the government is attempting to make it available. RU 486 is taken by a pregnant female during the first nine weeks of pregnancy under the supervision of a health-care professional. It causes the lining of the uterus, along with the embryo, to leave the uterus.

You may wonder why anyone would choose to have an abortion or take an abortion pill. There are many reasons why a female or a couple might want or need to end a pregnancy:

- The female has an illness or inherited disease that makes the pregnancy or birth dangerous to her health and might even cause her death.
- A test shows that the fetus is carrying a serious inherited disease or a serious birth defect.
- The mother or father is sick and unable to take care of a baby.
- The parents do not have enough money or time to take good care of a baby or they already have children and cannot afford another child.
- The parents feel they are too young to take care of a baby in a responsible manner.
- The female feels she was not ready to became pregnant.
- The female was forced to have sexual intercourse against her will—raped—and became pregnant as a result.
- The female is single and feels she is not able to raise a child on her own.
- The female did not intend or want to become pregnant.

People have very strong feelings about whether or not a female has the right to choose to have an abortion. In some countries, abortion is a right for all women and girls; in others, the right to abortion is either restricted or prohibited.

In 1973, the Supreme Court of the United States, which is the highest and most powerful court in the nation, ruled that a woman has the right to end an unwanted pregnancy. This ruling also says that no state can limit that right until very late in the pregnancy when the fetus could survive outside the womb. At this point, a woman can have an abortion only when her health or life is at risk.

The name of this Supreme Court decision is *Roe versus Wade.* Some individuals and groups are strongly for this decision and others are strongly against it.

People who support the Supreme Court decision call themselves "pro-choice." They favor a woman's right to choose for herself whether or not to have an abortion. They believe that this is a deeply private and personal choice and should therefore be made by the individual female, not by the government.

The people who believe that this decision should be changed call themselves "pro-life." They believe that the ruling allowing a woman to choose for herself whether or not to have an abortion is wrong. They believe that life begins when a baby is conceived and that an embryo or fetus has a right to life—a right to grow in the mother's body and to be born whether or not the mother wants to have a baby.

The rulings and laws about a woman's right to have an abortion have changed over the years and may continue to change. In 1992, the Supreme Court ruled to support their earlier 1973 decision guaranteeing a woman's right to abortion. However, the Court also ruled that any state in the nation can impose some reasonable restrictions on a woman's right to an abortion, but that it cannot outlaw abortion completely.

For example, some states require that before an abortion can be performed,

- any female under the age of eighteen has to have the consent of one or both of her parents or a judge's permission, depending on the laws of the state.

- a female has to be told about alternatives to abortion, such as continuing the pregnancy and either keeping the baby and becoming a parent or giving the baby up for adoption.

- a female must first meet with a health-care professional about having an abortion and then wait twenty-four hours before having one.

- the doctor or clinic must keep a detailed written record of all abortions performed.

Because laws can and do change, you might want to ask your parents or teacher what the laws and rulings about abortion are at this time, or what they are in your state.

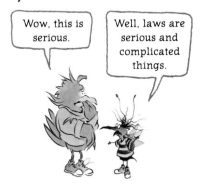

Wow, this is serious.

Well, laws are serious and complicated things.

Sometimes, usually during the early months of pregnancy, an abortion happens by itself, without a medical procedure. This is called a spontaneous abortion or a miscarriage. When this happens, the embryo or fetus is released from the mother's uterus without warning, often because it is not developing normally. Doctors do not always understand why miscarriages happen, but they know that females who have miscarriages can usually become pregnant again and give birth to healthy babies. The same is true for females who have chosen to have an abortion.

Part 6
Staying Healthy

25
Talk about It
Sexual Abuse

It's sad but true that some people's sexual behavior can be dangerous and even hurt others. This kind of behavior is called sexual abuse.

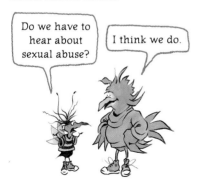

Do we have to hear about sexual abuse?

I think we do.

Sexual abuse is a subject that kids and adults find very hard and painful to think about and talk about. People often hear a lot of wrong and confusing things about it.

Though most kids have probably heard the words *sexual abuse,* that doesn't mean they know exactly what these words mean. *Sexual* means *having something to do with sex. Abuse* means *to treat wrongly, to mistreat.*

Sexual abuse happens when someone mistreats a person in a sexual way. It happens when someone who is more powerful than another person takes advantage of that person in a sexual way. It is wrong for anyone to take advantage of another person just because he or she is more powerful.

Most of us—kids and grown-ups—are taught rules as we are growing up about treating others with respect. Sexual abuse happens when someone breaks the rules that have to do with another person's body.

It happens when someone touches or does something to the private parts—the sexual parts—of another person's body that that person does not want him or her to do, or when someone makes another person touch or do something to his or her private parts that the person does not want to do.

This someone can be someone the person knows, someone the person loves, or a stranger. The truth is that it is most likely someone the person knows. Sexual abuse can happen between kids and adults—even between a parent and a child. It can also happen between one kid and another kid and between brothers and sisters. It can happen to both boys and girls.

The usual and normal daily hugging, kissing, touching, and holding hands that go on among

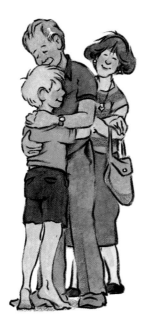

family members and good friends because they care about each other are not sexual abuse. A doctor's or nurse's physical examination of a person's body is not sexual abuse either. Everyone needs to have regular medical checkups to stay healthy.

Sexual abuse can feel painful or even hurt a lot. But not all sexual abuse hurts. In fact, a person can be abused in a way that can feel loving and gentle. When this happens, a person can feel very confused, because it's almost impossible to understand how something so wrong can feel gentle or loving.

Whether sexual abuse hurts or feels gentle or even loving, it is always wrong. People, especially grown-ups, know it is wrong. It is not your fault if it happens to you. Even if kids do not know the

rules, grown-ups do or should know the rules.

It is important always to remember that your body belongs to you. It's also important to know there are lots of people around who do care about kids and want to keep them safe.

If anyone tries to do something to your body that you don't want them to do or don't think they should do, say, "NO!" or "STOP!" or "DON'T!" to the person who is abusing you.

Some of you may have heard the word *harass*. *Harass* means *to annoy* or *bother*. If anyone harasses you—that is, bothers you—by talking about sex, by using rude or dirty words about sex when you don't want them to, or by talking about your body in a way that you don't like—tell that person to STOP! Even though that person is not actually touching your body, talking about sex or your body in this way can be a kind of sexual abuse.

There are some secrets with a trusted friend that are OK to

keep. But don't keep sexual abuse a secret if it happens to you or to a friend—even if someone tells you to keep it a secret.

Tell another person you know and trust—right away!

If the first person you tell doesn't listen to you, tell a second person. Talk about it until you find someone who understands **you** and believes you. That person will help you.

Always remember, if someone abuses you, it is NEVER your fault!

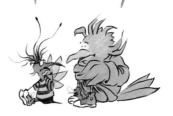

It's scary and creepy to hear about sexual abuse.

Yes, it is. But I do feel better just talking about it.

You also should never abuse anyone in any way. It's not fair. It's not your right. When someone says no to you, you must believe that person and honor that person's wishes.

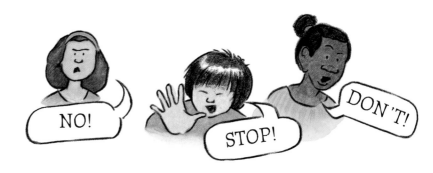

NO!

STOP!

DON'T!

Most people don't like to talk about sexual abuse, but now more people are talking about it. A kid can talk about it with a parent or friend or teacher. Very often it helps to talk with a school counselor, a social worker, a doctor, or a nurse—people specially trained to help. When a person who has been sexually abused can talk about it with someone he or she trusts, he or she may eventually feel better about it.

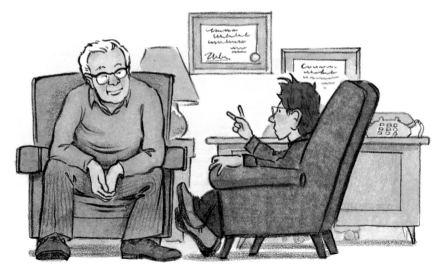

26
Checkup
Sexually Transmitted Diseases

Sex is usually a healthy, natural, and perfectly normal part of life. But sometimes sexual activities can be unhealthy.

Sexually transmitted diseases—called STDs for short—are diseases, infections, or illnesses that can spread from one person to another through sexual contact, from sexual touching to sexual intercourse. Another term for *STDs* is *STIs*—short for *sexually transmitted infections*. An older term for *STDs* is *VDs*—short for *venereal diseases*.

Infections and diseases such as colds and flus are caused by germs, which are so tiny they can be seen only by looking under a microscope. Not all germs cause sickness. But some, such as viruses and bacteria, do. Germs can be passed from one person to another by all sorts of contact—such as sneezing, shaking hands, and using the same glass, plate, or silverware.

STDs are different from most other infections—different from colds or the flu—because they are spread by sexual contact. Most people do not like to talk about STDs.

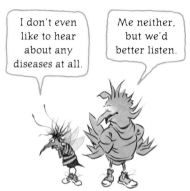

I don't even like to hear about any diseases at all.

Me neither, but we'd better listen.

There are many STDs. Some are not very serious. Others can be extremely serious; they can cause people not to be able to conceive a baby; they can even cause death. But many can be cured. And there are medicines and treatments that can make a person feel better if he or she has one of the STDs that cannot be cured.

Germs are not the only way a person can get an STD. A few STDs, such as pubic lice and scabies, are caused by tiny bugs.

Pubic lice are a fairly common STD. You may have heard people call lice "crabs." That's because lice are tiny six-legged bugs that look like crabs. Pubic lice like to live in warm, hairy spots, like the pubic area, and are passed on through sexual contact. Pubic lice can be easily cured by putting a medicine, which kills the lice, on the pubic area. These lice are different from common head lice, because head lice are not transmitted from one person to another by sexual contact. Head lice are not an STD.

Scabies can be, but is not always, an STD. It is caused by tiny bugs called mites that can cause severe itching in the areas around a person's genitals, as well as other parts of the body, except the neck and head. Scabies can be treated by putting medicine on the infected area.

Sexual contact is not the only way a person can get lice or scabies; contact with an infected person's sheets, towels, or clothing can also pass them on.

Syphilis, gonorrhea, and chlamydia are three STDs that are caused by bacteria. They can usually be cured by going to a doctor or a clinic and taking the correct medicine. However, if these STDs are not treated, a person can become very sick and lose his or her sight or the ability to have children. A mother who has one of these STDs can pass it on and cause damage to her newborn baby. Syphilis is an extremely dangerous STD, and if not treated can result in death.

Hepatitis B is an STD caused by a virus that infects the liver. Hepatitis B is very contagious and can be passed on by kissing, sexual intercourse, and unclean needles and syringes. People who take illegal drugs by using or sharing unclean needles and syringes run a big risk of getting hepatitis B. If you have your ears pierced or get a tattoo, you must make sure that a brand-new, germ-free needle is used. There is no cure for hepatitis B, but there is a vaccine that can keep a person from getting the virus. Most people who have this virus get well, but it can result in death.

Genital warts are another STD caused by a virus. Genital warts appear on a person's genitals or around the anus and can be extremely itchy and sore. Removal is the only treatment, but genital warts are very contagious and can grow back again. There is no cure for this STD. If the warts are not removed by a doctor, they can multiply quickly. Having genital warts can increase a female's risk of cancer of the cervix.

Herpes simplex virus causes an infection that can be, but is not always, sexually transmitted. This virus is passed from one person to another by skin-to-skin contact and is extremely contagious. There are two types of herpes simplex viruses. Herpes 1 causes blisterlike sores to form on or near a person's lips, mouth, nose, and eyes. Herpes 2, or genital herpes, causes blisterlike sores to form on or near a person's genitals and anus. No cure has been found for the herpes simplex virus, but both types can be treated by a doctor with medicine that can make the sores go away and make the infected area feel better. However, the sores can come back.

It is mostly adults and teenagers who get STDs. If a person has sexual contact, using a latex or polyurethane condom correctly and every time can help protect him or her from getting or passing on some of these infections. This is one way of practicing safer sex. Unprotected sex is extremely risky.

Not all infections are caused by sexual contact. But if a person feels discomfort or pain on or near any of the sexual parts of his or her body, it is important

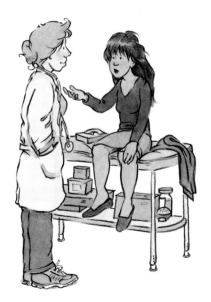

to tell his or her parents, the school nurse, or another trusted adult, so that a medical checkup can be arranged. If a person has a sexually transmitted disease, getting prompt medical care may not only make that person feel better, it may also save his or her life, as well as stop the spread of the infection to another person.

27
Scientists Working Day and Night
HIV and AIDS

HIV infection is the newest STD and the most dangerous of all sexually transmitted diseases. HIV is the germ—the virus—that causes AIDS.

The letters in the word *HIV* stand for *human immunodeficiency virus*—the scientific term for HIV. *Virus* means *a type of germ that can cause a person to become sick*. The letters in the word *AIDS* stand for *acquired immunodeficiency syndrome*—the scientific term for AIDS. *Acquired* means *something you can get*.

Immunodeficiency means *not able to protect against or fight infection*. *Syndrome* means *a group of symptoms or conditions that may accompany an illness or a disease*, such as a fever or loss of appetite.

What these words mean is that when people who are infected with HIV develop AIDS and become sick, their bodies are no longer able to protect against or fight infections. At this time, scientists and doctors believe that almost everyone who is infected with HIV will eventually

develop the symptoms or conditions of AIDS, such as coughing, fevers, weight loss, swollen glands, diarrhea, and being unable to think or see clearly.

A person who has HIV infection may not get sick for a long time, but almost everyone who develops AIDS eventually dies from one or more of its symptoms or conditions. At this time, there is no cure for AIDS, although there are some medicines and treatments that can slow down the virus.

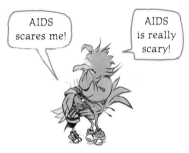

AIDS scares me!

AIDS is really scary!

Anyone can get HIV infection—young or old, male or female, rich or poor, heterosexual or homosexual, famous or not famous, weak or strong. Any person of any race or any religion can get infected with HIV and can develop AIDS. HIV infection has nothing to do with who you are; it can have a lot to do with what you do.

A blood test that doctors and nurses perform shows whether a person has been infected with HIV. If a person has the virus, he or she could remain healthy, even look healthy, and lead a good and productive life for many years. Without the blood test, it is not easy to know if the virus is in a person's body. The term *HIV positive* means that a person has HIV infection in his or her body.

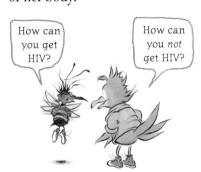

How can you get HIV?

How can you *not* get HIV?

Ways you cannot get HIV infection

• You cannot get HIV by playing tag, wrestling, hugging, shaking hands, giving a kiss hello, or giving a high-five to a person who has HIV.

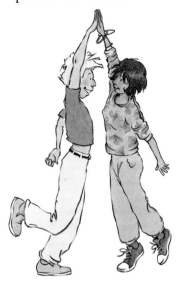

• You cannot get HIV from food, a plate, a comb, a brush, a doorknob, or a toilet seat that a person with HIV has touched.
• You cannot catch HIV the way you catch a cold, because the germ or virus does not travel through the air. That means you cannot get HIV from a cough or a sneeze.
• You cannot get HIV by donating blood.
• You cannot get HIV from a mosquito or a flea bite.
• You cannot get HIV just by being in the same room with someone who has HIV. That means that you cannot get HIV just by going to school with someone who has HIV.

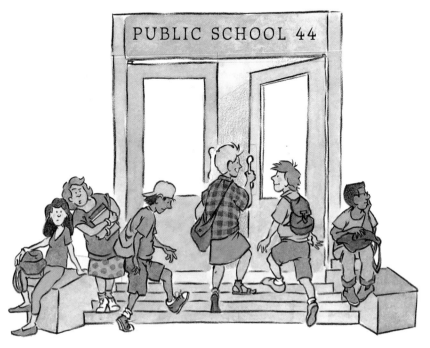

PUBLIC SCHOOL 44

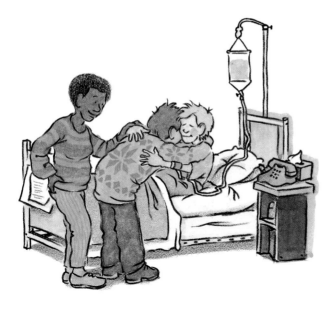

- You cannot get HIV from visiting someone who has HIV at his or her home or in the hospital.

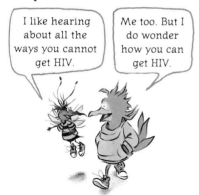

> I like hearing about all the ways you cannot get HIV.

> Me too. But I do wonder how you can get HIV.

Ways you can get HIV infection

- You can get HIV from a person who has the virus either from semen from the male's penis or fluids from the female's vagina. These body fluids carry HIV. That means you can get HIV from having sexual intercourse with a person who is infected with the virus even if that person appears to be healthy.

- It also means that if a person has sex involving the penis and the vagina, or the penis and the anus, or the mouth and the genitals, with someone who has HIV, and does not protect himself or herself correctly and every time, there is a real risk of getting infected with HIV.

  If a person chooses to have sex, using a latex or polyurethane condom with a water-based lubricant can help protect him or her from getting HIV. Unprotected sex is extremely risky.

- You can get HIV from the blood of a person who has the virus. That means you can get it if the blood from a person infected with HIV enters your bloodstream. However, all blood donated for kids, babies, and adults who need blood in a hospital or at home is tested to make sure it does not have HIV in it before it is given to them.

- You can get HIV if you take drugs and use a needle and syringe that has been used by a person who has HIV. People who take illegal drugs by using unclean needles and syringes or sharing needles run a big risk of getting HIV.

  But every time you get a shot from your doctor or nurse to keep you healthy, a brand-new, disposable, germfree, sterile needle and syringe are used and then thrown away in a safe place. You cannot get HIV from brand-new, germfree needles and syringes. If you have your ears pierced or get a tattoo, you must make sure that the needle used is brand-new, germfree, and disposable.

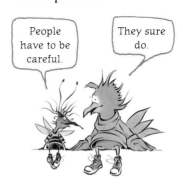

> People have to be careful.

> They sure do.

- A female who is infected with HIV and has the virus when she becomes pregnant can pass it on to her baby while it is in her uterus or during birth. That is why some babies are born infected with the virus. And some mothers who are infected with the virus can pass it on to their babies through their breast milk.

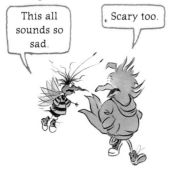

This all sounds so sad.

, Scary too.

Luckily, scientists and doctors have discovered ways in which people can protect themselves from getting HIV and lessen their chances of developing AIDS. One way is to abstain from having sexual intercourse with another person. This is called abstinence and is the only fully safe way people can protect themselves from getting HIV through sexual contact.

If a person chooses to have sexual intercourse, using a latex or polyurethane condom can lessen his or her chance of getting HIV infection. You may have heard the term "safer sex." Using a latex or polyurethane condom correctly and every time is one way people are practicing safer sex. Not sharing needles is

another way to avoid the chance of getting HIV infection.

Scientists all over the world are working day and night in laboratories to try to make a vaccine that will prevent a person from being infected with HIV if he or she comes into contact with it. Just as there are vaccines to protect people from being infected with measles, mumps, or polio, an HIV vaccine could prevent a person from being infected with HIV and developing AIDS.

Scientists are also working on making pills, shots, or other treatments that they hope will help people who already have the AIDS virus to lead longer and

healthier lives. They hope that such treatments will either keep the virus quiet so that it will not be able to harm a person or will eliminate the virus from a person's body entirely.

But even without a vaccine or treatment, people can help protect themselves from getting HIV infection by knowing how the virus is passed from one person to another.

Many people who are HIV positive or who have developed AIDS are able to go to work or school and carry on with most parts of their lives for a number of years, until the virus makes them too sick.

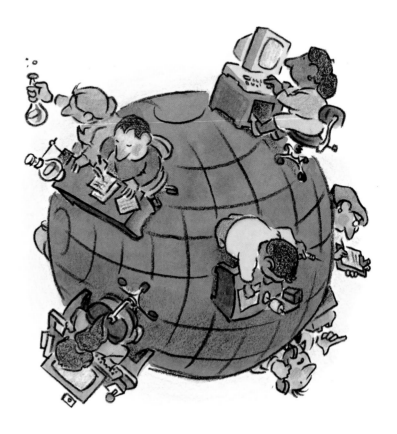

And yet people, both kids and adults, who are HIV positive or who have developed AIDS have been discriminated against. Some children, along with their families, have been forced to move to new neighborhoods or cities in order to go to school, and some adults have lost their jobs and been forced to move—only because they are HIV positive or have developed AIDS.

Having HIV infection as well as developing AIDS is sad and painful in many ways. So, if you know someone who is HIV positive or has developed AIDS, treat that person kindly. Shake hands, say hello, give a hug, talk with that person, laugh and even cry with that person, and work and play with that person—all these things are safe to do—and treat that person as you would treat any good friend.

28
Staying Healthy
Responsible Choices

A large part of growing up is learning to take care of yourself in a healthy way.

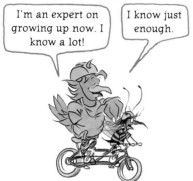

I'm an expert on growing up now. I know a lot!

I know just enough.

Eating healthy foods, exercising almost daily, keeping your body clean, wearing clean clothes, staying away from drugs and alcohol, and having regular medical checkups—all of these things can help you be healthy and stay healthy as you go through puberty.

But there's more to staying healthy than just taking good care of your body. It also means taking responsibility for your own actions—for yourself and for what you do. It means making healthy choices for yourself,

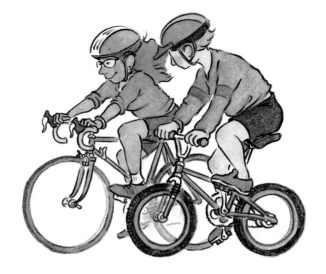

including choices about your body and about sex. And it means having respect for yourself and your own decisions.

Staying healthy also involves having healthy relationships with other people. That means not only taking good care of yourself, but taking good care of your friends—both boys and girls. Having a good friend or friends as

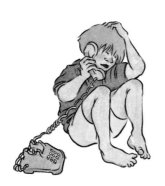

you grow up can help you learn how to have healthy relationships with other people that involve sharing, caring, and respect for others as well as for yourself.

As you go through life, friendship—being a good friend—is a big part of every healthy relationship, whether two people like each other a lot, or love each other a lot, or like and love each other a lot.

Yet puberty is a time when friends, even good friends, often try to persuade or pressure each other to try out new things. Some of these things, which may involve sex, alcohol, or drugs, may be things you do not want to do, or are not ready to do, or are

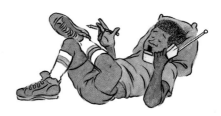

afraid to do, or feel it is not safe to do. That's when it's important to make the decision that is best for you—one that is safe and healthy for you.

Everyone makes mistakes and has bad judgment once in a while, and you probably will too. But most of the time, you can and will make responsible choices—ones that are good for you, right for you, and healthy for you and your friends.

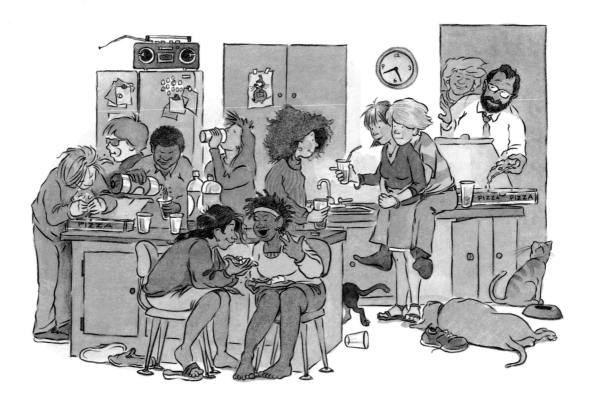

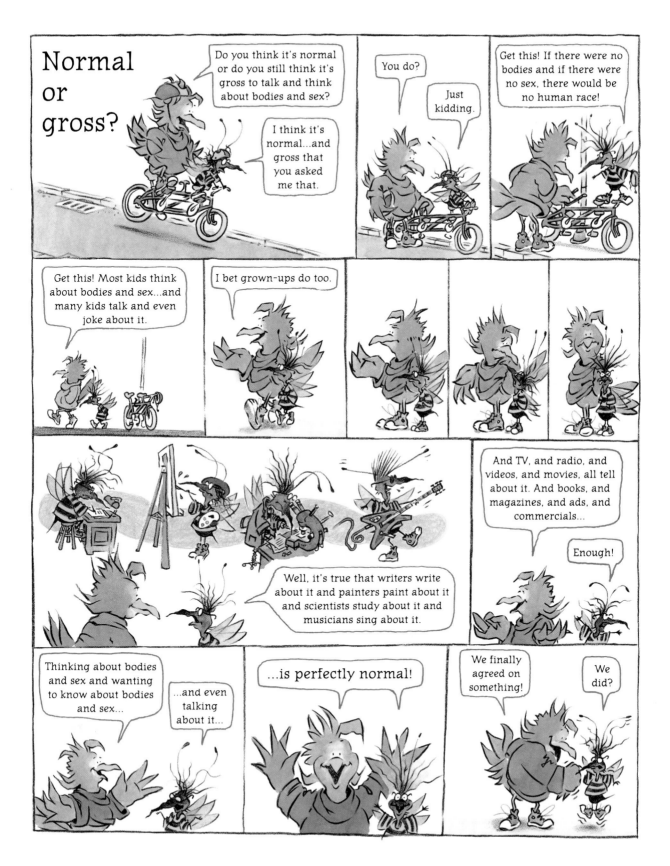

Thank You!

We could not have written and illustrated this book without the help of the following old and new friends and colleagues. Some of them read the whole manuscript; others read only a chapter. Some read the manuscript once, others read it numerous times. Many helped with the drawings. Everyone had something to say about this book, and everyone answered any question we had, often more than once. The people listed here all have one thing in common. They care deeply about the health and well-being of children and have enormous respect for children.

RHH and ME

Deb Allen, elementary school science coordinator and teacher, The Devotion School, Brookline, Massachusetts

Tina Alu, sexuality education coordinator, Cambridge Family Planning, Cambridge, Massachusetts

Joanne Amico, health educator, Pierce School, Brookline, Massachusetts

Bonnie S. Anderson, Ph.D., professor of history, Brooklyn College, Brooklyn, New York

Fran Basch, professional trainer, Planned Parenthood League of Massachusetts, Cambridge, Massachusetts

Merton Bernfield, M.D., Clement A. Smith Professor of Pediatrics, director, Joint Program in Neonatology, Children's Hospital, Boston, Massachusetts

Sarah Birss, M.D., child psychiatrist, developmental pediatrician, Cambridge, Massachusetts

Larry Boggess, school administrator, writer, Richmond, Indiana

Alice Miller Bregman, senior editor, New York, New York

Rosa Casamassima, consultant, Medford, Massachusetts

Deborah Chamberlain, parent, Norwood, Massachusetts

David S. Chapin, M.D., director of gynecology, Beth Israel Hospital, Boston, Massachusetts

Chuck Collins, parent, San Francisco, California

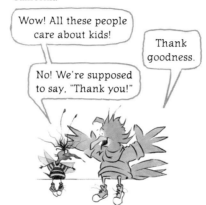

Edward J. Collins, M.D., assistant clinical professor, University of California at San Francisco, California

Julia Collins, student, San Francisco, California

Paula Collins, parent, San Francisco, California

Sara Collins, student, San Francisco, California

Sally Crissman, science educator, Shady Hill School, Cambridge, Massachusetts

Mollianne Cunniff, health educator, Brookline Public Schools, Brookline, Massachusetts

Kirsten Dahl, Ph.D., associate professor, Yale University Child Study Center, New Haven, Connecticut

Mary Dominguez, science teacher, Shady Hill School, Cambridge, Massachusetts

Catherine Donagher, parent, Brookline, Massachusetts

Sheila Donelan, teacher, M.E., Fitzgerald School, Cambridge, Massachusetts

Sandra Downes, teacher, Amos E. Lawrence School, Brookline, Massachusetts

Nancy Drooker, sexuality education consultant, San Francisco, California

Nicki Nichols Gamble, executive director, Planned Parenthood League of Massachusetts, Cambridge, Massachusetts

Frieda Garcia, president, United South End Settlements, Boston, Massachusetts

Judith Gardner, Ph.D., psychologist, Brandeis University, Waltham, Massachusetts

Trudy Goodman, M.Ed., child and family therapist, Cambridge, Massachusetts

Ben Harris, student, Cambridge, Massachusetts

Bill Harris, parent, Cambridge, Massachusetts

David Harris, student, Cambridge, Massachusetts

William Haseltine, Ph.D., chief, Division of Human Retrovirology, Harvard Medical School, Dana Farber Cancer Institute, Boston, Massachusetts

Gerald Hass, M.D., pediatrician, Cambridge, Massachusetts; physician in chief, South End Community Health Center, Boston, Massachusetts

M. Peter Heilbrun, M.D., chairman,

Department of Neurosurgery, University of Utah, Salt Lake City, Utah

Robyn O. Heilbrun, parent, Salt Lake City, Utah

Doris B. Held, M.Ed., psychotherapist, Harvard Medical School, member of the Governor's Commission on Gay and Lesbian Youth for the Commonwealth of Massachusetts, Cambridge, Massachusetts

Michael Iskowitz, chief counsel for poverty, AIDS, and family policy, U.S. Senate Committee on Labor and Human Resources, Washington, D.C.

Chris Jagmin, designer, Watertown, Massachusetts

Larry Kessler, executive director, AIDS Action Committee of Massachusetts, Boston, Massachusetts, commissioner, U.S. National Commission on AIDS, Washington, D.C.

Robert A. King, M.D., assistant professor of child psychiatry, Yale University Child Study Center, New Haven, Connecticut

Antoinette E. M. Leoney, Esq., parent, Salem, Massachusetts

Elizabeth A. Levy, children's book author, New York, New York

Jay Levy, M.D., professor of medicine, Cancer Research Institute, University of California School of Medicine at San Francisco, California

Leroy Lewis, teacher, Martin Luther King School, Cambridge, Massachusetts

Carol Lynch, director of counseling, Planned Parenthood Clinic, Brookline, Massachusetts

Lyn Marshall, teacher, The Atrium School, Watertown, Massachusetts

Kristin Mercer, student, Arlington, Massachusetts

Ted Mermin, teacher, The Atrium School, Watertown, Massachusetts

Ronald James Moglia, Ed.D., director, Graduate Program in Human Sexuality, New York University, New York, New York

Rory Jay Morton, teacher, Shady Hill School, Cambridge, Massachusetts

Eli Newberger, M.D., director, Family Development Program, Children's Hospital, Boston, Massachusetts

Brenda O'Conner, teacher, M. E. Fitzgerald School, Cambridge, Massachusetts

Dian Olson, educator and trainer, Planned Parenthood League of Massachusetts, Cambridge, Massachusetts

June E. Osborn, M.D., dean, School of Public Health, University of Michigan; chairman, U.S. National Commission on AIDS, Washington, D.C.

Jimmy Parziale, teacher, Michael Driscoll School, Brookline, Massachusetts

Kyle Pruett, M.D., clinical professor of psychiatry, Yale University Child Study Center, New Haven, Connecticut

Jeffrey Pudney, Ph.D., research associate, Harvard Medical School, Boston, Massachusetts

Jennifer Quest-Stern, student, Cambridge, Massachusetts

Louise Rice, R. N., associate director of education, AIDS Action Committee of Massachusetts, Boston, Massachusetts

Sukey Rosenbaum, parent, New York, New York

Kate Seeger, teacher, Shady Hill School, Cambridge, Massachusetts

Rachel Skvirsky, Ph.D., associate professor of biology, University of Massachusetts, Boston, Massachusetts

Paula Stahl, Ed.D., executive director, Children's Charter Trauma Clinic, Waltham, Massachusetts

Michael G. Thompson, Ph.D., child psychologist, Cambridge, Massachusetts

Laurence H. Tribe, Tyler Professor of Constitutional Law, Harvard Law School, Cambridge, Massachusetts

Maeve Visser Knoth, librarian, Cambridge Public Library, Cambridge, Massachusetts

Polly Wagner, teacher, The Atrium School, Watertown, Massachusetts

Lilla Waltch, author, Cambridge, Massachusetts

Rosalind M. Weir, parent, Cambridge, Massachusetts

Ilyon Woo, student, Cambridge, Massachusetts

Donna Yee, Ph.D., consultant, Visions Inc., Cambridge, Massachusetts

Barry Zuckerman, M.D., professor of pediatrics, Boston University School of Medicine, Boston, Massachusetts

Pamela Zuckerman, M.D., pediatrician, Boston, Massachusetts

A special thank you to our editor Amy Ehrlich for her wholehearted commitment to this book and her courage for taking it on, to our art director Virginia Evans for listening to us and seeing our vision, to our associate editor Jane Snyder for keeping track of every word and everyone, to their colleagues at Candlewick Press for their enthusiastic support, to our agent Elaine Markson for her friendship and belief in this book, and to our designer Lance Hidy for his wonderful eye.

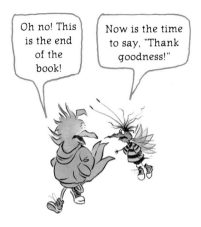

Oh no! This is the end of the book!

Now is the time to say, "Thank goodness!"

Index